The Research Publishing Playbook

Jeff Choi

The Research Publishing Playbook

Springer

Jeff Choi
Surgery
Mass General Brigham
Boston, MA, USA

ISBN 978-3-032-28503-4 ISBN 978-3-032-28504-1 (eBook)
https://doi.org/10.1007/978-3-032-28504-1

This Springer imprint is published by the registered company Springer Nature Switzerland AG
The registered company address is: Gewerbestrasse 11, 6330 Cham, Switzerland

With sincere gratitude to my mentors and mentees, to whom I credit all lessons

Preface

Peer-reviewed manuscripts dominate the academic currency, shaping everything from graduate school admissions to faculty promotions and grant funding. Many researchers receive formal training on the technical ingredients of good research—bench techniques, statistical methods, and other foundational skills. However, the *process* of envisioning an idea, recruiting and motivating a team to complete a project, communicating findings effectively, and convincing editors and reviewers that a manuscript deserves publication, is a hidden curriculum often relegated to individual mentors or personal trial and error.

The process *of taking a research idea to a peer-reviewed publication is a distinct skill set that requires deliberate practice.* Mastering this skill set liberates more time for scientific inquiry and facilitates translating research activity into productivity.

This book provides concise, actionable guidance on optimizing every step of the publication journey, from idea conception to the "accepted for publication" notification. It covers practical strategies that are not covered in most classrooms, including file organization and team management strategies, designing effective figures and tables, avoiding prevalent study design pitfalls, and perfecting cover letters and response to reviewers. I hope this book can help learners in any discipline master the hidden curriculum of publishing manuscripts and bypass years of avoidable inefficiency.

This is *The Research Publishing Playbook.*

Boston, MA, USA — Jeff Choi

Contents

Part III After the Writing

About the Author

Jeff Choi is a trauma and acute care surgeon at Mass General Brigham and faculty at Harvard Medical School. He is a surgeon-data scientist trained at Stanford University, where he completed medical school, graduate training in epidemiology and biomedical informatics, general surgery residency, and surgical critical care fellowship. He has authored over 100 peer-reviewed publications in leading journals, including *JAMA*, *JAMA Surgery*, and *Annals of Surgery*.

He has mentored students and trainees across multiple institutions, helping many achieve their first or high-impact publications. He was the founding instructor for Stanford School of Medicine's "Practical Introduction to Research Skills," a course designed to systematically teach efficient academic productivity. His work focuses on building reproducible systems that transform research ideas into tangible, publishable outputs.

Part I
Before the Writing

Chapter 1
Foundations of Research Efficiency

Optimize the Research Project Workflow

Most research projects follow a linear sequence from idea conception to manuscript submission. This approach is logical, but inefficient. Shifting from serial to a parallel workflow is the key to consistent productivity (Fig. 1.1).

Assemble a research team Whenever possible, a research project is best conducted as a team. The right team can accelerate the project timeline and allow multiple projects to run in parallel. Effective team members share three traits: ***passion*** for the project, a ***skillset*** that adds value, and ***time*** to contribute to the project. Missing any of these elements leads to disengagement, and disengagement is contagious. With a balanced group of experienced team members, new learners can be integrated within and amplify the team. Teaching and elevating trainees is a core academic responsibility and should not be sidelined for the sake of speed.

Start writing the manuscript early Many researchers begin manuscript writing only after completing experiments or analyses. This delays progress unnecessarily. Large portions of a manuscript—background and research aim, study design and analytic plan, summary of existing literature, and methodologic limitations—can be completed before any data collection begins (Fig. 1.1). Writing is iterative and often becomes the rate-limiting step of the research project lifecycle, especially for researchers whose primary training is not in writing. Start writing the manuscript as soon as possible and revise continuously as the project evolves.

Manage concurrent research projects A principal investigator who understands team members' skill sets, constraints (e.g., vacations, exam weeks), and the actual workload required to complete each project should be able to manage multiple projects at once (Fig. 1.2).

J. Choi, *The Research Publishing Playbook*,
https://doi.org/10.1007/978-3-032-28504-1_1

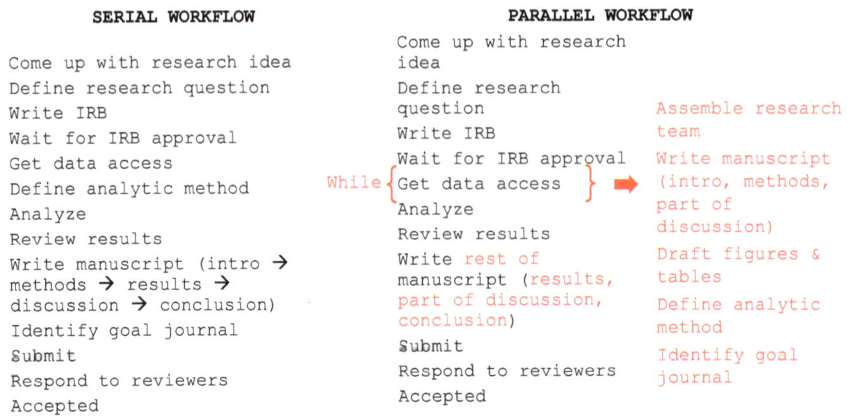

Fig. 1.1 Serial vs parallel project workflow. Typical research projects follow a linear sequence of tasks. A parallel workflow can improve the research team's efficiency

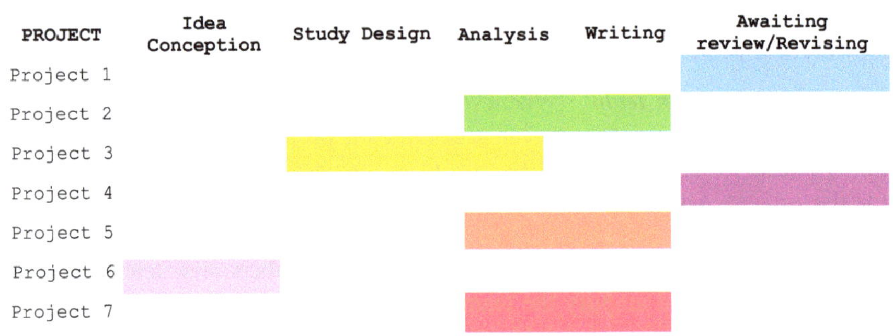

Fig. 1.2 Project portfolio of a multi-project principal investigator. An effective principal investigator should manage multiple research projects at different stages, reallocating priorities and resources as needed to sustain momentum within the research group

Most projects naturally experience periods of rapid progress and slowdown due to logistical delays or external demands. An effective multi-project principal investigator should reallocate priorities and resources across projects to sustain momentum across the entire research group. If one project is expected to stall over particular dates, the pace of another project should be adjusted to make strong headway in the interval. For example, while a trainee finetunes the final manuscript draft for one project, a second should be undergoing intensive manuscript draft revisions, a third undergoing data analysis, and another, undergoing study design.

The multi-project principal investigator should aim to generate tangible outputs and provide actionable feedback every week to ensure at least one project moves forward. This approach allows you to control the rate-limiting steps of every project across your entire portfolio.

Solidify Productive Habits

Identify and reclaim wasted time Most of us waste more time than we realize. Every time an email or phone notification breaks concentration, our brain requires time to readjust to the task at hand. Some studies estimate that over a third of a workday is wasted due to task switching. It is not uncommon for wandering thoughts to interrupt our workflow:

Did I respond to that email from my colleague a couple of *days ago?*
When was that potluck dinner I was invited to again?

Many valuable minutes are often disregarded in the morning while half-awake in bed, or at night while scrolling on our phones. These small losses accumulate. Reclaiming and repurposing precious time for research every day could mean the difference between never having time for research and consistent productivity.

Over 1 week, use a stopwatch to quantify your baseline wasted time each day: how long you can stay focused before your mind drifts and how much time is lost to task-switching. The results are usually sobering. Most of us only sustain true focus for minutes, or even seconds. Reclaiming even 15 min of wasted time each day adds up to over 90 h in a year—roughly two full weeks of research time.

Commit time to research every day Research is rarely a leading daily priority and falls to the wayside among competing professional and personal demands. Without consistent commitment, research stalls. Once lost, momentum is challenging to recover.

Regardless of other commitments, time must be committed to research every day. Much like eating meals or showering, research—be it conducting experiments, reading relevant literature, or designing new studies—must become an inseparable daily routine. We must become rewired so that a day without some time dedicated to research—even if for 5 min—must be made to feel incomplete. The optimal time to dedicate to research may vary, depending on the research task and personal preferences. For example, you may code best in the evenings and write better in the mornings. You may need at least an hour of block time to code, but can write manuscripts in short bursts of several minutes if needed. You may realize that you can review or revise no more than one full manuscript draft a day. Through trial and error, establish a daily research schedule that fits your natural rhythms and the demands of different tasks. Consistency is the only reliable path to sustained productivity.

Stay focused Multitasking is inefficient. The brain cannot execute two meaningful tasks simultaneously: we can walk while holding casual conversations, but we cannot meaningfully participate in an online meeting while also reviewing a grant application. Indeed, low-cognitive-burden tasks such as simple data extraction may occur with background distractions, but most research tasks demand focus. During protected research time, notifications should be silenced and our undivided attention tuned to the one task at hand.

The length of time we can sustain focus varies, and it should be measured and extended. The Pomodoro technique—working intensely for a defined duration followed by a timed interval—is one useful way to ensure every minute dedicated to research counts. For example, start a timer when you begin a task. Stop it the moment your attention drifts—when you find yourself checking social media, your email, or thinking about unrelated plans. Repeat this exercise to establish your baseline, then extend this interval intentionally. Once your focus duration plateaus, use this interval as your standard work block and schedule breaks around it.

For further strategies, *The One Thing* and *Atomic Habits* provide useful frameworks for building durable, productive routines.

Document and Organize Systematically

Many project folders devolve into a jumble of files such as "manuscript_v6," "dataset_final," and "dataset_finalfinal." Upon request for revisions months after submission, teams waste hours trying to track down the true final dataset, manuscript draft, or the analytic code that produced the results. The research project should be organized such that years after its completion, anyone can open the project folder and trace a clear path from the raw data to the final manuscript.

Use subfolders systematically Each project should have its own main folder with subfolders delineating key contents, such as "dataset," "analysis," "figures_and_tables," "manuscript," and "revisions." An "old_files" subfolder can host outdated files to keep active folders clean.

Manuscripts often cycle through multiple journals, each with different formatting requirements. Content submitted to each journal should be hosted under separate subfolders. If the manuscript is rejected, this subfolder should be moved to the "old_files" subfolder.

A "readme" document in the main project folder can summarize key changes made across file versions or document essential notes regarding the project. Using the same folder structure across all projects facilitates maintaining a predictable workflow. Consistency breeds efficiency.

Annotate coding files When conducting data analysis in R, SAS, STATA, or another programming language, the ideal code file should be able to process the raw dataset and generate every result, figure, and table in the manuscript with a single run. Annotating code files is critical for collaboration for interpreting your own work months later when revision requests arrive. For example, key analytic sections should be labeled (e.g., data preprocessing, sensitivity analysis) and reasons for important analytic decisions should be documented within the code file (e.g., specific exclusion criteria, regression model of choice; Fig. 1.3).

```
#### This script will calculate TROUT (trauma frailty outcomes) Index scores##
###input: data frame containing ICD10 codes as column value
### outout: TROUT INDEX score. Optional TROUT INDEX frailty risk strata

####packages ####
library(dplyr)
library(tidyr)
library(data.table)

#function identify only first 3 characters of ICD10 codes
first3<-function(x) {substr(x,start=1,stop=3)}

#keep only first  3 characters of ICD10 codes  within dataframe
#columns containing ICD10 codes  titled "I10_DX..." i.e. I10_DX1, I10_DX2,...
df <- df %>%
  mutate_at(vars(contains("I10_DX")),first3) %>%
  mutate_at(vars(contains("I10_DX")),as.factor)
```

Fig. 1.3 Annotated code file. Coding files should be organized and annotated to allow any reader to reproduce all relevant study results and figures starting from the original dataset. The logic behind key decisions can also be noted directly on the coding file as a reminder

Manual edits to datasets, such as changing numbers in an Excel sheet, are strongly discouraged. Manual changes are error-prone and make it challenging to trace or correct errors. Instead, a research team should adopt a shared common programming language and make all dataset modifications using fully annotated code, ensuring every change is traceable.

Standardize file naming conventions File names should follow a standardized naming convention that facilitates both analysis and easy identification. Many programming languages are case sensitive; using lower-case letters and designating spaces with an underscore ("_") simplifies calling files for analysis. For example, rather than "Rodent Population Project Data.csv," a file titled "rodent_population_project_data.csv" may be easier to call on a coding file.

A standardized naming convention, such as "projectname_filetype_date" facilitates rapid file identification. For example, compare two files named "Manuscript version 6" and "manuscript final final version." Is "final final version" newer than "version 6"? Moreover, without opening each file—which wastes time unnecessarily—it may be unclear which project they belong to. The confusion only grows if a revision is requested months after submission or when a team member who did not create the original files must take over revisions.

Instead, files named "readmissions_after_trauma_manuscript_10062023" and "readmissions_after_trauma_manuscript_10132023" are instantly distinguishable. Both clearly pertain to a project regarding readmissions after trauma, and the file ending in "10132023" (October 13th, 2023) is more recent than the one ending in "10062023" (October 6th, 2023).

Figure 1.4 illustrates the suboptimal versus the optimal research project file organization scheme.

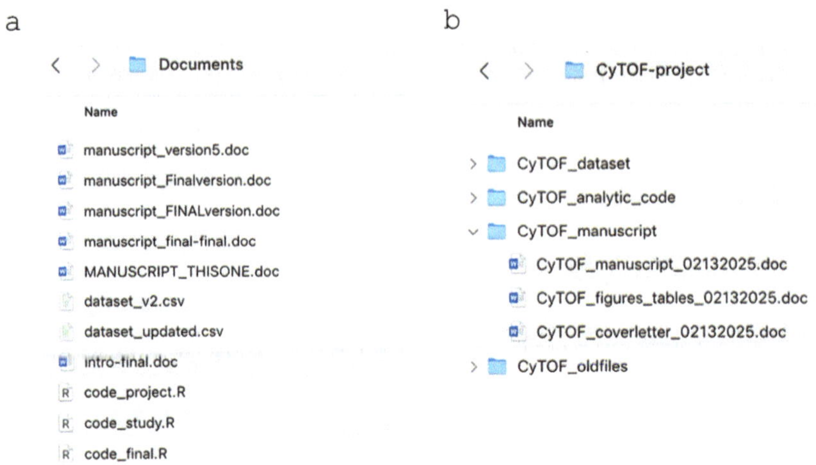

Fig. 1.4 Research project folder organization. (**a**) Suboptimal organization. Various files, potentially from multiple projects, are stored in a generic "Documents" folder. Each file must be opened to determine its content; (**b**) Optimal organization. Each research project is hosted in a dedicated folder. Outdated materials are archived in an "old files" subfolder, while current files are stored in clearly labeled subfolders and named to immediately convey the content

Back up files All project data should be backed up regularly to both the cloud and an external hard drive. The biggest setback to productivity would be losing data and having to start a project over from scratch. Nearly 20 years later, I still remember seeing a desperate sign taped to the hallway of a research building where I worked in high school: "Computer stolen, entire PhD work inside." Back up your data. Regularly.

Chapter 2
Essential Ingredients of High-Functioning Teams

Ingredients of Team-Building

Most projects are best undertaken as a team. Principal investigators recruiting team members must be savvy team managers with a clear understanding of (1) required skill sets, (2) projected timeline, and (3) essential resources.

The research team must collectively possess all skills needed to take the project from start to finish. Relying on a single member for a critical task (e.g., complex technical analysis) risks putting the entire project on standstill if that person were to become unavailable. People get sick, experience significant life events, or decide to leave the team—life happens. Building redundancy through overlapping expertise can protect against these disruptions. In clinical research, consulting an external statistician is common for rigorous study design and analysis, but external experts often are in high demand and often have competing commitments. Outsourcing pivotal tasks risks losing control of a project's timeline. Whenever possible, recruit a methodological expert to join the team as a fully integrated team member who can prioritize moving the project forward. Domain expertise alone is rarely sufficient to drive high-quality projects forward.

Grasping a realistic timeline for project completion is essential to recruit and retain team members. Misalignment between expected and actual timelines can breed dissatisfaction and disengagement. A project projected for 6 months during recruitment but stretching beyond a year may lose key members once they graduate or take on other commitments. Conversely, overestimating a short project as a year-long effort may deter talented members seeking shorter-term commitments. Grasping an accurate project timeline requires a detailed understanding of the project's demands and familiarity with similar work. Setting realistic expectations is critical to sustain engagement.

Principal investigators should ensure all resources necessary to complete a project are secured before assembling the full team. A strong team should not sit idle

J. Choi, *The Research Publishing Playbook*,
https://doi.org/10.1007/978-3-032-28504-1_2

while waiting for institutional review board approval, access to an essential database, or other logistic hurdles. These should be handled by the principal investigator and the lead member in advance. If target journals require article processing charges, funding should be arranged in advance.

Recruiting the Team

The resources have been secured. The project timeline and needed skill sets are clear. How do you recruit great team members?

Passion is insufficient Inquiry emails and first meetings often overflow with enthusiasm. Yet many principal investigators know this familiar pattern:

> A new member reaches out with excitement for an opportunity to join the group. They sign on for a project. Other team members orient the new member and teach technical skills. The new member is excited to read through the literature and learn about the project background. They stay engaged for a couple of weeks or months. Then an exam, vacation, or life event emerges, and contact becomes less frequent for a couple weeks. Meetings are missed, and deadlines slip, but I tried to be understanding. Progress resumes with some apology, until another competing event emerges. The cycle repeats, until momentum disappears and the once-enthusiastic recruit is now MIA.

This is a predictable and an avoidable setback. Passion is insufficient to sustain engagement. For most members, a research project is not a top life priority. Many are juggling other professional or personal commitments and still fine-tuning their sustainable bandwidth of commitments. A research project is often one of the first commitments to be dropped among more pressing, tangible commitments, such as exams and applications. Recruiting members based on passion alone leads to high turnover and stalled projects.

How can you recruit a team member who will make meaningful contributions and stay engaged to the end? The ideal team member must have *growth objectives aligned* with the project, have *a relevant skillset* to contribute meaningfully, and have a *willingness to prioritize* the project (Fig. 2.1).

Aligned growth objectives Every prospective team member has a personal motivation for reaching out. Some may have a niche interest in the specific project, a general interest in the research domain, or need research experience for career advancement. Each member's motivation must be unpacked into concrete growth objectives.

The principal investigator and prospective team member should use frameworks such as SMART (specific, measurable, achievable, relevant, and time-bound) to ensure that growth objectives can be met by the specific project. A member with clear growth objectives aligned with a project, even if their subject-matter interest is modest, is more likely to see a project through than someone with deep subject

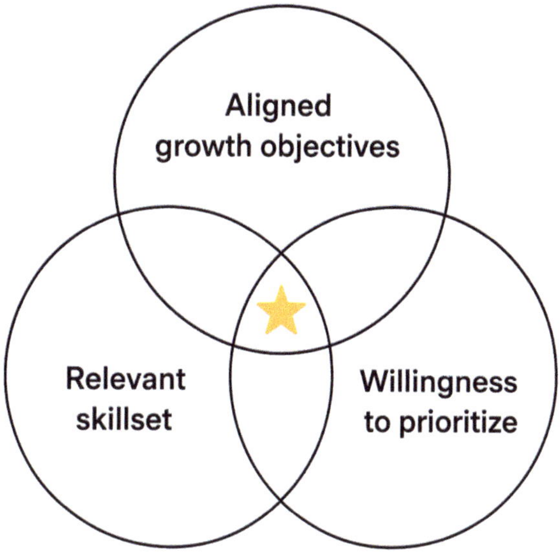

Fig. 2.1 Characteristics of an ideal research team member. Passion alone is insufficient to sustain long-term engagement to the end of a project

interest but no focused plan for their own development. Alignment is the foundation of engagement.

Skillset No one member needs to have all the skills required to take a project from start to finish. Not all principal investigators are experts in every task needed to complete a project. Like the general manager assembling a sports team, the principal investigator must ensure that the collective team skillset covers all tasks needed for project completion.

Renowned principal investigators, like general managers of top professional sports teams, may be able to choose among many interested experts for every needed project task. Most principal investigators are not in this position. Even for well-established groups, welcoming and teaching new trainees is valuable and a necessary duty. Some members may contribute primarily through their willingness to learn and grit. It is the principal investigator's job to ensure that every project has an appropriate balance of senior and new members to ensure there is (1) adequate collective team skillset to carry a project to completion, (2) bandwidth for senior members to teach and supervise, and (3) not so many new members that growth opportunities become diluted (Fig. 2.2).

Willingness to prioritize Time is not the true constraint; priority is. Everyone has the same 24 h a day and faces fluctuating commitments and life events. What drives the perseverance to see a project through is the willingness to *prioritize* a project in spite of other commitments.

After discussing growth objectives and assessing skill fit, the principal investigator should ask directly:

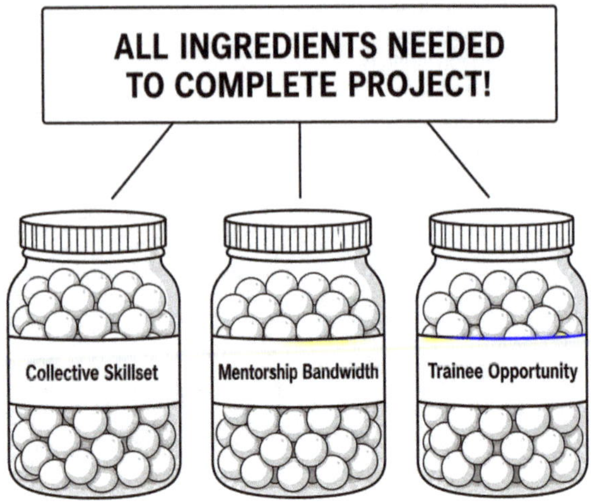

Fig. 2.2 Essential "skill" ingredients for a research project. The team as a whole must have all the skillsets needed to complete a project. A right balance of senior and new members is needed to ensure bandwidth for teaching and opportunity for growth

> Given everything we have discussed, are you willing to prioritize this project at this stage of your life?

Rather than an immediate verbal commitment, request written confirmation by email within a few days of the introductory meeting. A written commitment is more enduring and allows time for reflection. Remember, losing members mid-project is costly. Upfront commitment is essential.

Set reasonable hurdles Well-established principal investigators may receive many inquiries to join their teams. It may not be feasible to meet with every prospective member to gauge their fit and commitment. Reasonable pre-meeting requirements—such as submitting a curriculum vitae and a brief paragraph outlining their interest and goals—can filter out those unwilling to follow through on basic tasks or sending mass inquiry emails. If someone cannot meet this minimal expectation, they are unlikely to stay engaged with a project and its challenges through completion.

Joining a Team

Prospective members should be just as deliberate about choosing a research team as principal investigators are about recruiting. The earlier story of the disengaged trainee may look very different from the trainee's perspective:

> I heard about Professor A's research and reached out. I had little research experience, but the research seemed exciting, so I decided to join the group and learn. My first task was to "read the literature," but no one gave clear directions. At the first few weekly lab meetings, I didn't have much to report other than that I was reading. A senior member was assigned to teach me how to run an experiment, and after a couple of weeks, I could do it independently. Then I had exams and spring break, so I let my senior member know, who said it was fine

to be away for a couple of weeks. I didn't think I needed to tell Professor A directly, who, I'm sure, has more important concerns. While on spring break, Professor A emailed asking about progress. I wondered whether I made a mistake by not notifying them, but I made good progress after returning from break. However, Professor A was traveling frequently, and it was challenging to find time to meet. My main contact was the senior member, but they were also busy with their own work. Over time, I became unsure whether my efforts would translate to a publication or whether I was being helpful at all in the lab. Eventually, I decided research wasn't for me.

Just as principal investigators must recruit reliable members, prospective members must join labs with the infrastructure, leadership, and mentoring capacity to help them grow and drive projects to the finish line. Indeed, a prominent principal investigator has a high probability of having the infrastructure and experience to provide an enriching experience for the team and be academically productive. However, not every lab is a good fit for everyone at every stage of their career. Like in professional sports, dynasties rise and fall. How do you pick a winning team?

Mentoring track record Principal investigators who have mentored trainees to peer-reviewed publications are likely to continue being successful mentors. "Success" here is defined narrowly: guiding trainees to complete peer-reviewed publications. This is not the only measure of mentorship quality, but it is the most relevant for a book focused on finishing projects.

Trainees who want to ensure their research activity translates to productivity should query the following:

How many publications has the prospective mentor published as senior author (the last listed author), with a trainee first author?

How many trainees have produced multiple first-author publications with the prospective mentor?

A principal investigator who has helped several trainees publish multiple first-author publications is likely to have found a reproducible mentoring process. However, lack of such a track record should not disqualify early-career investigators; everyone starts with an empty mentoring track record. Early-career investigators often provide more personal, hands-on mentorship, and joining a winning team early can pay dividends.

Research track record A prospective mentor's publication record—often visible on lab webpages, institutional profiles, or Google Scholar—is far more than a list of publications. It offers valuable insight into how their team operates and what opportunities a trainee can expect.

The pattern of collaborators may show whether projects are driven by a tightly contained core team or by a collaborative multi-institutional network. The former may offer consistent guidance and well-controlled project timelines yet may focus on narrower scientific scopes with fewer opportunities to engage diverse experts. The latter may offer access to broader resources, yet authorship roles may be less predictable and multi-site projects often move more slowly.

Patterns in authorship can reveal whether trainees routinely lead projects or whether opportunities concentrate around a select few. The pace and consistency of publications may reveal general timelines for projects and whether infrastructure that supports productivity is stable, declining, or accelerating. Multiple publications using certain methods or datasets may suggest a reproducible pipeline and established standard operating procedures that new members can plug into. Finally, the prospective mentor's own trainee-era publications may indicate whether they have hands-on mastery of specific technical skills or primarily have domain expertise with experience coaching technically skilled team members. Taken together, these patterns can help trainees evaluate whether a lab's structure, resources, and pace aligns with their goals.

Leadership style The principal investigator is responsible for ensuring projects cross the finish line. Every mentor is different in how they motivate teams to achieve this aim, and trainees must uncover their own preferences.

Do you prefer working with a pace-setter, who will set hard deadlines and check in regularly to ensure milestones are not missed, or someone who grants more freedom to work at your own pace? Do you prefer a mentor who gives direct instructions on how to solve specific problems or one who expects you to troubleshoot independently? What are nonnegotiables traits for you in a mentor?

A mentor perfect for one trainee may be a poor fit for another. Finding the right mentor requires first clarifying your own working style and a clear assessment of how the mentor leads.

Expectation-Setting

The mentor has identified a strong addition to the team—someone whose growth objectives align with the project, who brings valuable skills, and who is willing to prioritize the project. The trainee has reviewed the mentor's track records and leadership style and decides the fit is right. Before beginning the project, two common reasons mentor-mentee relationships break down must be addressed: authorship and momentum (Fig. 2.3).

Authorship Authorship expectations must be explicit, consistent, and documented at the outset. Disputes about authorship eligibility or order incite damaging conflicts within teams, and often arise because expectations were not clarified.

The principal investigator must clarify the standards to be listed as an author. For example, if a member contributes to a project over several months but leaves the group before the manuscript is drafted, how much should they have contributed to be an eligible coauthor? What if they leave because the project stalled through no fault of their own? These questions must be addressed proactively using fair, consistent, and measurable expectations. For example, for a member recruited to help

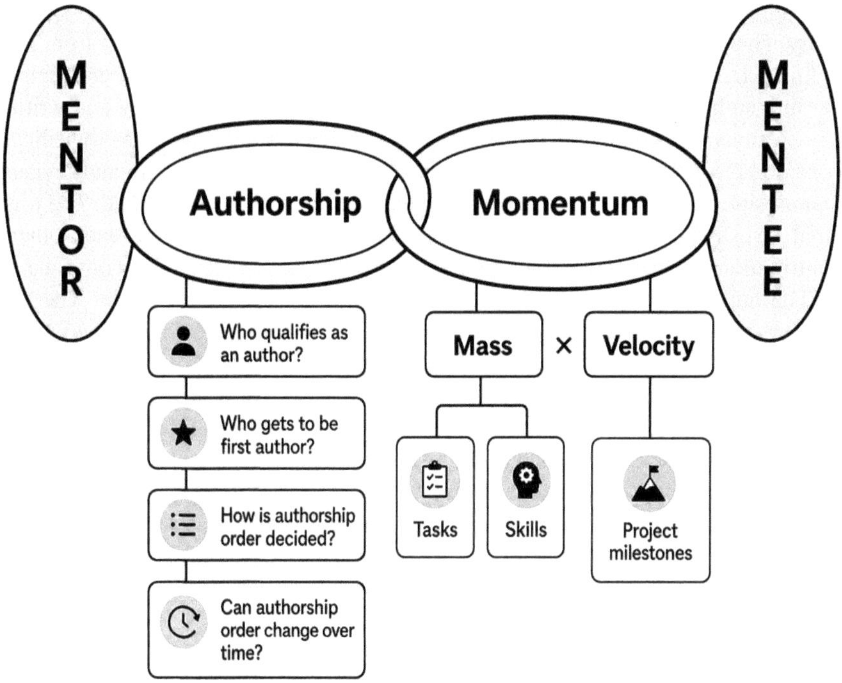

Fig. 2.3 Common reasons mentor-mentee relationships break down. Misaligned expectations regarding authorship, including qualifications and author order, are a frequent source of conflict and must be explicitly defined at the beginning of every project. Relationships also deteriorate when projects lose momentum. The principal investigator must identify all essential tasks for project completion and ensure the team collectively possesses the skills to complete these tasks. Predefined milestones must be met on schedule

interview subjects for a mixed methods study, the minimum number of interviews to complete could be an author eligibility criterion.

The International Committee of Medical Journal Editors recommends that authors meet all four criteria:

1. *Substantial contributions to the conception or design of the work; or the acquisition, analysis, or interpretation of data for the work*
2. *Drafting the work or reviewing it critically for important intellectual content*
3. *Final approval of the version to be published*
4. *Agreement to be accountable for all aspects of the work in ensuring that questions related to the accuracy or integrity of any part of the work are appropriately investigated and resolved.*

These criteria effectively require each author to have ownership of a measurable component of a project. Importantly, authorship should not be offered as a political favor. Even if unchallenged, such practices will be noted by the team, erode trust, and damage the principal investigator's reputation for fairness.

Authorship order should reflect the magnitude of contribution to the specific study. The first author should have done the most to advance the project from start to finish. In larger teams, much of this work may be invisible to others. For example, the first author may have spent considerable time designing the study and writing key portions of the manuscript before other members joined, and plans to dedicate considerable time responding to reviewers. Responding to reviewers and revising manuscripts is a key responsibility of the author that is often overlooked. The principal investigator must ensure that every team member is aware of each other's contributions so that authorship order decisions are transparent and uncontested.

The authorship order can change throughout a project's life cycle. The first author is typically designated at the study outset, yet their actual contribution may turn out to be less than another team member's due to competing demands or failure to meet expected timelines. As soon as it is apparent that a change in authorship order is warranted, the principal investigator should meet with affected team members to explain the rationale and seek agreement. Of note, sometimes, two members may truly contribute equally and substantially to a project. Many journals recognize co-first authorships and members can list their own names first on their respective curriculum vitae, with co-first authorship noted.

Authorship expectations and order should be communicated in writing. Setting the authorship order is the principal investigator's responsibility. Delegating this to the team invites resentment and misunderstanding, as individual members rarely see the full landscape of contributions.

Momentum A second common failure point for mentor-mentee relationships is loss of momentum. A research project is rarely a trainee's top priority and is easily displaced by competing personal and professional demands. The team should come to a mutual consensus on the expected momentum that should be sustained throughout the project lifecycle. A simple framework is helpful for unpacking pitfalls:

$$\text{Momentum} = \text{mass} \times \text{velocity}$$

"Mass" is the total set of tasks required to complete the project. Projects can slow or fail when the team lacks the collective skillset to execute necessary tasks, the principal investigator misjudges the technical demands of the study, or a trainee is assigned work beyond their experience without sufficient support. To ensure adequate mass, the principal investigator must fully understand the study design, its methodologic requirements, and team members' skill sets.

"Velocity" is the speed at which major project milestones are met. A project should be divided into clear, time-bound milestones, and internal deadlines must be held to the same standard as grant funding or conference abstract deadlines. When one deadline is missed without consequence, it sets a precedent, and subsequent deadlines become easier to miss. A series of missed deadlines degrades momentum, and once lost, momentum is difficult to recover. Many projects never make it to publication because the principal investigator fails to set a realistic but firm pace and allows delays to become the norm.

Parting Ways with Grace

Despite best efforts, there may be times when a principal investigator or member decides the partnership should end. A principal investigator may feel that the member has become a "ghost", lacks time or motivation to stay engaged, or is slowing a project to the point of degrading momentum. No one benefits from forcing work on someone who no longer wishes to participate. Likewise, a trainee may feel that the team lacks direction, the project is stalled, or their efforts are better invested elsewhere. Many of these situations arise not from misconduct but from misaligned expectations, priorities, or timing.

Once the decision is made, the separation should be handled professionally. With time and reflection, emotions fade, and the value of even small contributions or lessons learned from the partnership becomes clearer. Rather than assigning blame, it is better to explain that continued collaboration is not the right fit at this moment, express appreciation for the effort contributed, and part on good terms with clear communication regarding any authorship eligibility. A graceful exit preserves reputations, protects future opportunities, and reflects professionalism expected in academic research.

Chapter 3
The Manuscript Roadmap and Danger Zones

You have solidified productive habits, assembled a high-functioning team, and aligned expectations. Before diving into the mechanics of data analysis, figure preparation, or manuscript drafting, all team members must understand the roadmap of manuscript acceptance and danger zones that derail projects. The scientific merit of a study is essential but is insufficient for manuscript acceptance. The art of presenting a clear, compelling story to the right audience at the right time is just as important. Knowing common danger zones that derail projects can ensure the team avoids mistakes that waste months of effort and threaten momentum.

The Manuscript Roadmap

Submitting a manuscript is not the finish line. It is closer to the halfway mark. Once submitted, a manuscript typically undergoes several sequential evaluations, each with its own failure points (Fig. 3.1).

The corresponding author is typically either the first author or the principal investigator and will be responsible for responding promptly to journal communications and any queries after manuscript publication (e.g., readers' request for data). The typical post-submission roadmap for a manuscript is as follows:

1. **Editorial quality control**. Journal editorial staff first screen for formatting (e.g., bibliography) and policy compliance (e.g., blinding).
2. **The editor's desk**. The reviewing editor may be the editor-in-chief or one of several editors who can adjudicate submissions. At this stage, a manuscript can either be rejected ("desk reject") or sent out for peer review. Particular articles in select journals, such as invited articles, may be accepted for publication directly by the adjudicating editor, but this is rare for typical original research. Following a desk reject, the submission process repeats with another journal.

J. Choi, *The Research Publishing Playbook*,
https://doi.org/10.1007/978-3-032-28504-1_3

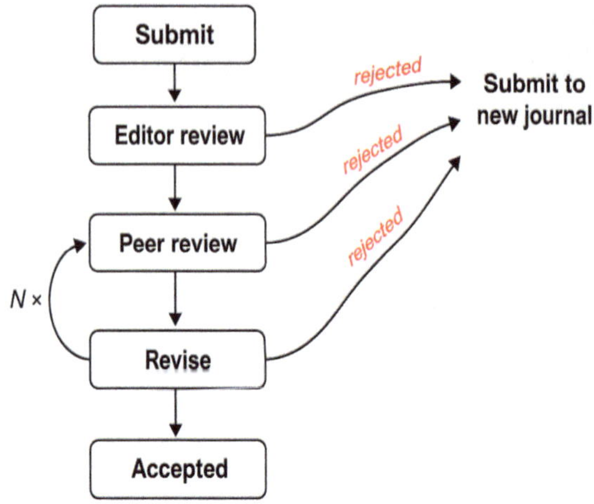

Fig. 3.1 Points at which a submitted manuscript can get rejected. A manuscript may be rejected at the editor's desk before peer review, following initial peer review, or at any subsequent round of revisions

3. **Peer reviewer selection**. If the editor decides to send the manuscript out for peer review, the editor must secure qualified peer reviewers. This step alone may take weeks or months. Ideal peer reviewers are domain or methodologic experts who can provide a critical, unbiased review of the study's rigor and potential impact. Each journal has policies governing the minimum number of peer reviewers (typically at least two) and whether they are blinded to the submitting authors.
4. **Peer review**. Reviewers are typically given a timeframe within which to review and make a recommendation, along with comments regarding the manuscript. The review timeframe and the rigor with which this is enforced are variable. If a reviewer fails to submit a recommendation despite weeks of nudging, the editor may begin the search for a new reviewer to fulfill the minimum number of reviewers before adjudicating a decision.

   If reviewers disagree strongly, another reviewer may be invited for additional perspective.
5. **Editorial decision**. Once enough adequate reviews are obtained, the editor (or a group of editors) deliberates and issues a decision: typically, "minor revision," "major revision," "reject," or, rarely, "accept."
6. **Revisions by authors**. A revision opportunity does not guarantee eventual acceptance. Authors are given a specified time to respond to reviewer comments and revise their manuscript.
7. **Rereview**. Upon receiving the response to reviewers and revised manuscript, the editor may formally accept the manuscript (e.g., if reviewers requested very minor revisions and all were clearly addressed) or send the manuscript out for rereview to the original or new reviewers. Reviewers may recommend acceptance (if satisfied with the response and revisions), further revision (if the authors were close to but did not fulfill important requests), or rejection (if dissatisfied with the response).
8. **Final decision**. The second round of recommendations is received by the editor, who may issue a final decision or request another set of revisions. At least one or two revision cycles should be expected before acceptance.

The journey after manuscript submission often spans several months. The timeline expands quickly if the manuscript is rejected across multiple journals. Each rejection after peer review, and even desk rejection, consumes weeks or months. Failure to target the appropriate journal is costly.

Editors and Peer Reviewers

To understand the path to manuscript acceptance, we must next understand the decision-makers: editors and peer reviewers.

Most journals have an editorial board that includes an editor-in-chief, editors who can adjudicate manuscripts, a managing editor who oversees day-to-day operations, and additional board members who provide strategic guidance. Some journals assign editors to specific article types, such as "innovations," "brief reports," or "perspectives." Some journals also have statistical editors who review study design or analytic rigor, typically upon reviewer or editor request.

Journal editors are accomplished academics with established expertise in fields relevant to the journal. Most editors volunteer their time to the journal. This critical point bears repetition. Most editors volunteer their time.

While a few journals may employ salaried editors-in-chief or offer modest honoraria, the majority of editors manage full-time academic careers alongside their editorial responsibilities. Impatient emails seeking an adjudication within a month of initial submission are ill-advised. Journals often publish expected timelines (e.g., average weeks to first decision), and these should be respected. Only substantial deviations from published norms warrant a polite query, and the timing of such queries should be decided carefully by the principal investigator.

Peer reviewers are selected by editors for their content or methodological expertise, and similarly volunteer their time. For some submissions, an editor may know several trusted reviewers—colleagues, reliable prior peer reviewers, or well-known experts. For others, an editor may need to search more extensively by consulting colleagues, journal reviewer directories, or publication records (e.g., authors cited in the submission). Selected reviewers receive an invitation email and typically have a few days to accept their invitation.

Some journals request that authors suggest potential reviewers during submission. It is inappropriate to suggest close colleagues in hopes of obtaining favorable reviews. While identifying unbiased experts may be challenging in niche domains, authors must make a genuine effort to recommend reviewers without conflicts of interest.

While a recognition of expertise and some would argue, a duty among academics, peer review is uncompensated work that must be balanced against other professional commitments. Many academics receive multiple peer review invitations each week. Reviewers may prioritize requests from journals aligned with their field or society memberships, from editors they know personally, or for manuscripts that pique their interest. Some may accept invitations from prestigious journals because ad hoc reviewing for such journals is itself professionally valuable.

Editors continue sending reviewer invitations until enough reviewers accept to meet the journal's minimum threshold. Because motivations and the availability of reviewers vary, the process of securing reviewers can be slow.

Peer Reviewers Are Not Your Enemy

After a series of frustrating rejections, and especially after receiving comments that seem misguided or unfair, it may be tempting to view peer reviewers as obstacles standing between you and your manuscript's publication. This attitude must be abandoned. Peer reviewers are truly peers who volunteer their time, offer external insights, and suggest improvements, even if the ultimate recommendation is a rejection. Indeed, some peer reviewers may have biases or misunderstand points despite best efforts. Some comments may feel rude. Not all peer reviewers are trained in offering constructive feedback, and not all journals enjoy a deep bench of seasoned expert reviewers. This reality does not diminish the value of the peer review process.

We must remember the ultimate purpose of writing a manuscript: communicate findings clearly to advance a field. Reviewers are your first readers. If they misinterpret a finding, the writing must be clarified for future readers. If they challenge your conclusions, more convincing data or narrative is needed. If criticisms feel unfair, treat them as opportunities to engage in professional, evidence-based dialogue. Peer reviewers should be perceived as tough coaches—sometimes mistaken, but ultimately, committed to shaping your manuscript into the best possible form before it enters the public domain.

Recall that editors and peer reviewers volunteer their time alongside their full-time jobs. Many review manuscripts late at night, on weekends, or during time that could be spent with family (Fig. 3.2).

Make their jobs as easy as possible. Keep the manuscript crystal-clear and succinct. Grammatical errors, sloppy formatting, or ambiguous writing, tax the reviewer's cognitive bandwidth and render a positive evaluation less likely.

An important note: Peer reviewers may have authored key studies you cite. Missing or misinterpreting seminal work can damage the submission's credibility. A thorough, up-to-date literature review is critical. If you point out limitations of prior studies, ensure that critiques are factual, measured, and professional. Your reviewer may have authored these studies, and antagonizing them would be unwise.

Targeting the Right Journal

Editors aim to publish high-quality submissions that will be well-read by their readership, cited frequently, and advance their field. Many journals publicize key metrics such as editorial desk rejection rate, overall acceptance rate, and average time to initial and final decisions. For the most reputable journals, acceptance rates may be less than 5%.

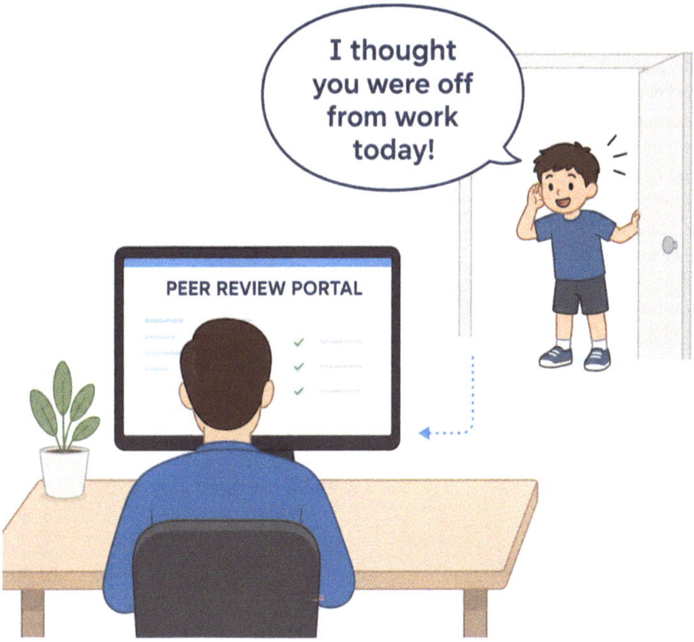
I thought you were off from work today!
PEER REVIEW PORTAL

Fig. 3.2 Make the peer reviewers' jobs as easy as possible. Peer reviewers volunteer their time

Each rejection adds considerable time to the publication process. Because manuscripts can be submitted to only one journal at a time, mis-targeting a journal can leave a completed manuscript without a home for months or even years. Some completed manuscripts never get published because momentum is lost after repeated rejections. Many principal investigators can attest to at least one orphaned manuscript sitting in an old hard drive. Proper journal targeting is essential to protect time, team morale, and productivity.

Strategies to find appropriate targets Most researchers are aware of the hierarchy of journals within their domain. For example, flagship journals such as *Science, Nature, JAMA, and NEJM* represent the highest tier for many physician-scientists. Shooting for the stars—submitting to the most selective journals and sequentially working downward—is not a good strategy. The reality is, conducting world-class research is not possible for every research group, every time. A publication somewhere is better than a manuscript sitting unseen in a hard drive.

Every rejection has a cost. Besides the administrative work of reformatting submissions and waiting for reviews, repeated rejections increase the risk of getting scooped. If another group publishes a similar study first, your manuscript's novelty is lost, and the chances of finding a home become considerably lower. Editors and reviewers will question the incremental value of your study. The first to publish sets the narrative. Everyone else must justify their added value, and being late to a body of literature makes publication incrementally more challenging.

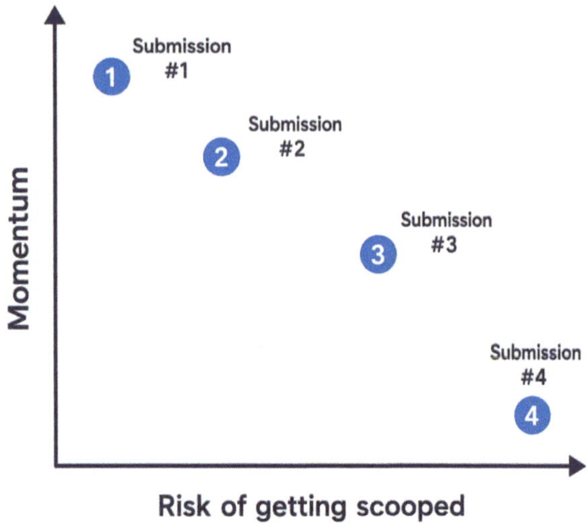

Fig. 3.3 The cost of failing to target the appropriate journal. Multiple revisions erode team momentum, prolong the time to publication, and increase the risk of getting scooped. Once a similar study is published, substantially greater effort is required to demonstrate incremental novelty and marginal value

Selecting the appropriate journal is analogous to selecting colleges to apply to. A manuscript has unique merits and limitations, akin to an applicant's portfolio. Not every manuscript is competitive at the top tier. Because simultaneous submissions are not permitted, refining the target journal list is critical. Submitting only to journals with low selectivity can limit visibility. Submitting only to unreasonable "reach" journals can waste time. Submitting to a short list of reasonably reachable journals may be worthwhile depending on expected turnover times, pace of competition, and team member's timelines (e.g., graduate school application deadline).

Several clues can help identify realistic journals. First, see where the cited literature was published. Journals that have repeatedly published studies you cite are likely aligned with the scope of your work. Second, review recently published articles from potential target journals. A journal that has not published on your particular topic for several years is unlikely to change course. A journal that prioritizes randomized controlled trials is unlikely to consider an observational study unless there is an exceptionally convincing story. The methodology section of recent articles is a good indicator of the level of study quality the journal typically accepts. Journals that routinely publish well-designed studies that fail to reject the null hypothesis likely value rigorous methodology over sensational findings.

The bottom line: do not shoot for the stars. Be pragmatic. Every rejection has a cost (Fig. 3.3).

With a thoughtful and realistic target list, every manuscript should find a home within a few submissions, where it can reach the right audience and achieve meaningful impact.

Beware of predatory journals After publishing as the corresponding author, your inbox will begin receiving messages such as:

> Dear esteemed Professor [your name], based on your exceptional expertise, we would like to invite you to contribute a manuscript to [Journal Name].

Most of these invitations come from predatory journals and should be ignored. These journals present themselves as legitimate yet exist primarily to profit from publication fees. They often lack genuine peer review, have minimal editorial oversight, and scrape corresponding author contacts to mass-solicit submissions with guaranteed acceptance. While legitimate journals occasionally solicit article submissions, particularly for invited commentaries or special issues, these invitations typically come from well-known editors to established investigators. Predatory solicitations are usually easy to spot. The journal's scope has no connection to your publication track record, and the email is excessively flattering.

Danger Zones that Undermine Acceptance

Methodologic rigor Rigorous methodology is the foundation of every research study. Seasoned reviewers often begin with the methods section; if the methodology is flawed, the subsequent results, discussion, and conclusion are irrelevant.

Every research project must involve a methodologic expert. Today, it is easy to download advanced statistical packages, learn how to interpret models online, or ask generative artificial intelligence models to write analytic code. Self-teaching study designs and analyses without direct guidance from a methodologic expert is like performing an operation by watching videos online. You may complete the operation, but complications will follow.

Unfortunately, suboptimal methodology is common in contemporary literature. Misunderstandings of foundational statistical concepts such as p-values (covered in a later chapter) have contributed to the scientific reproducibility crisis. With growing interest in applying machine learning techniques and accessibility to scripts that can apply complex algorithms using a few lines of code, many submissions showcase "novel algorithms" implemented by researchers with no formal training.

Many methodologically weak studies do continue to pass peer review. The reality is that, except for a handful of well-resourced journals, most editorial teams and peer reviewer pools lack sufficient methodological expertise to catch every error. The responsibility for protecting scientific integrity lies with individual researchers. Methodologic rigor is not an ideal to aim for but a requirement. Every study must involve a methodologic expert from the start.

Objective reporting Overselling findings is one of the quickest ways to invite rejection. From the title and abstract to the discussion and conclusion, the manuscript's tone should match the rigor of the study design, strength of the findings, and limitations inherent to the methods. Declarative titles such as "X causes Y" may sound attention-grabbing. However, unless the study design establishes causality beyond reasonable doubt, seasoned editors and peer reviewers will detect the overstatement.

It is natural for the research team to be deeply interested in their work. The study topic is exciting, the motivation obvious, the methodology sound, and the findings seem important. Enthusiasm for one's research is healthy, but editors and reviewers approach manuscripts as objective evaluators. They will not share the same level of enthusiasm about a study's importance or novelty without good reason. Language that overstates conclusions or reflects illogical or biased interpretations of findings will be poorly received. Instead, a tone of measured humility that acknowledges limitations and presents data-driven interpretations demonstrates scientific maturity.

Article type and brevity Most journals accept several types of manuscripts. Some categories are obvious and tied to the study design—scoping reviews, randomized controlled trials, or perspectives. Many journals offer full-length submissions (e.g., original article, original investigation) and abbreviated formats (e.g., brief report, research letter). Beyond formatting differences, both typically undergo the same review process and are publicized and indexed in the same fashion.

A full-length submission is not inherently more prestigious. The goal of publishing is to communicate research findings clearly to the right audience. If this objective can be accomplished using fewer words, the abbreviated format is often the better choice. Every word must be essential to communicating findings. Rather than padding to approximate word limitations, words should be trimmed aggressively at every opportunity to ensure concise communication.

Chapter 4
Understanding the Research Landscape and Managing Citations

A comprehensive literature review is essential to understand the research landscape, identify the knowledge gap your study will address, and contextualize your study findings. Woe to those who dedicate considerable time and resources to complete and submit a manuscript, only to have a reviewer comment that the exact study has been published by another group!

The Challenge of Information Overload

Many studies evaluate similar questions, and it is exceedingly rare for a single study to settle a research question definitively. The pendulum of evidence often swings. Take the example of appendicitis, one of the most common conditions that general surgeons manage. Nearly 300 years after the first appendectomy (operation to remove the appendix), debates surrounding the optimal management of this single pathology persist. Multiple randomized controlled trials continue to compare strategies across different populations and outcomes. Many surgeons can name one or two seminal appendicitis trials, but many other trials, and even more observational studies, go largely unnoticed. It is unrealistic for any surgeon to remain up to date on every nuanced evidence regarding the management of appendicitis. Given the same patient, surgeons' management will differ based on the particular subset of evidence they happen to know, their practice patterns, and their biases.

In surgery alone, over 300 articles are published each day, and this volume grows exponentially. Information overload is the reality of modern research (Fig. 4.1).

No researcher can claim a perfect literature review: the body of evidence is too formidable and ever-expanding. Likewise, no introduction or discussion section can fully capture the totality of existing evidence within a few hundred words.

J. Choi, *The Research Publishing Playbook*,
https://doi.org/10.1007/978-3-032-28504-1_4

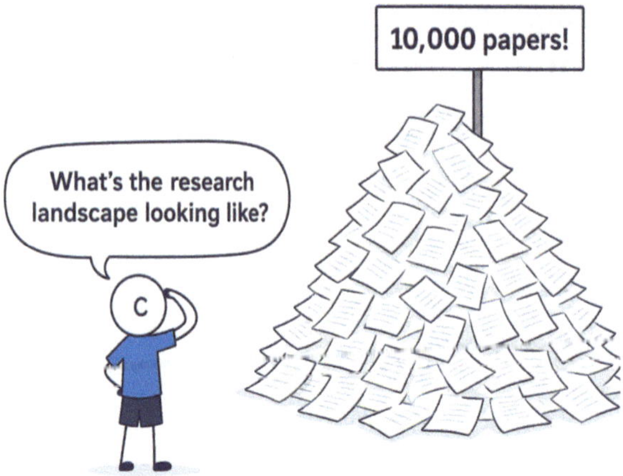
10,000 papers!
What's the research landscape looking like?
C

Fig. 4.1 Information overload in modern research

How to Practically Grasp the Research Landscape

Given this reality, how can a researcher navigate the vast research landscape, identify a meaningful question, and design a study that advances a field? From a trainee's perspective, experienced investigators seem to have an intuitive sense of knowledge gaps and pressing questions. Trainees often join a team after the study blueprint has been set and are told, "familiarize yourself with the literature."

No book can fully impart this intuition experienced investigators appear to possess. There is no bypassing years of reading, thinking, and conducting research. However, there are practical ways to start building habits that help better understand the research landscape.

Review articles within respected journals The first strategy is to read review articles published in the domain's most respected journals. Most journals publish unsolicited review articles, but a domain's most respected journals often invite leading experts to write them or publish only the highest-quality contemporary summaries. Simply typing "*review of [topic]*" into search engines often yields highly-cited articles, but highly-cited does not necessarily mean high-quality. Citations can accumulate due to search engine mechanics (e.g., keyword match) and the Matthew effect ("the rich get richer"). A better approach is to search for review articles directly within the most respected journals. High-quality review articles often provide a structured overview of the existing landscape and offer a mental map of established and emerging research areas.

References cited by high-quality review articles The references cited by high-quality review articles can inform the next set of articles to provide more in-depth context to specific subtopics. Reading every article from beginning to end and critiquing each in depth is usually impractical. Understanding the research landscape typically constitutes two aims:

1. Recognizing what important questions remain unanswered.
2. Learning how those questions could be answered.

The Limitations (typically within Discussion) and Methods sections offer the best sources to elucidate these aims.

Limitations section The limitations section often highlights unanswered questions. In the limitations, authors often discuss threats to the study's internal validity (i.e., accuracy of findings) or external validity (i.e., generalizability of findings) and propose directions for future studies. Rather than immersing in the information overload of what has already been done, studying the "limitations" can efficiently highlight what has not been done and how this could be done. Once a set of possible research directions comes to mind, a simple question can refine a focused study aim:

What is a critical and urgent knowledge gap in this field, and how would filling that gap advance the field forward?

Methods section Reviewing the Methods facilitates familiarity with resources (e.g., databases, cell lines, potential collaborators) and techniques (e.g., statistical, study design) available to address questions. The Methods form the foundation of every study. Becoming familiar with the Methods of high-quality studies is akin to assembling a survival toolkit before a trip into the wilderness. You don't know which tools will prove most useful, but the larger the toolkit, the more capable you will be to navigate any challenging scenario.

Conducting a Comprehensive Literature Review

Once you gain some understanding of the research landscape and identify a knowledge gap worth answering, a comprehensive literature review is needed for the specific study. Depending on your field, relevant sources may range from published articles, books, to artifacts. There are many search engines available, including arXiv, PubMed, Embase, Web of Science, Google Scholar, Scopus, and JSTOR. Newer search engines with artificial intelligence-enabled literature search continue to emerge. If you are affiliated with a higher-education institution, a research librarian can be invaluable in designing a thorough search strategy.

The following section will detail strategies for one of the most widely-referenced databases in biomedical research—the United States National Library of Medicine's PubMed. While specific search strategies may vary across search engines, the core principles of a structured search should be broadly applicable.

Effective Literature Search Using PubMed

The effective literature search should yield the relevant articles you are looking for. Understanding how content is archived within the search engine is critical to taking full advantage of search strategies.

PubMed is maintained by the US National Library of Medicine, a part of the National Institutes of Health. Journals that meet specific quality criteria are indexed on PubMed (i.e., their articles are aggregated on PubMed). Each article is deposited via automated pipelines along with structured metadata, including the article title, author names, affiliation, journal information, and keywords (often supplied by the authors at submission).

Many articles on PubMed are a part of MEDLINE, a curated collection of biomedical and life sciences journals. Articles indexed on MEDLINE are manually reviewed by US National Library of Medicine indexers who assign medical subject headings (MeSH) terms to each article. MeSH terms follow a publicly available hierarchy of controlled vocabulary that categorizes articles for efficient retrieval.

As an illustration, imagine that you are interested in studies related to placing a tube into the chest (chest tube) to remove blood that builds up in the chest cavity after traumatic injury (hemothorax). Searching "chest tube for hemothorax" will retrieve articles containing this or similar phrases anywhere in the record (e.g., title, abstract, keywords), regardless of context. Four simple tools can improve precision to retrieve articles you seek: field tags, wildcards, proximity search, and Boolean operators.

Field Tags Field tags restrict the search to specific metadata, such as the title, abstract, or MeSH terms. PubMed has many field tags, which can be called using square brackets (Table 4.1). The term of interest should precede the field tag.

For example, "chest tube for hemothorax[ti]" retrieves articles with the word "hemothorax" in the title; "English [la]" retrieves articles written in English; and "("2020"[dp]:"2024"[dp])" retrieves those published between 2020 and 2024.

MeSH terms are an especially powerful field tag because they capture standardized concepts. In our example, the MeSH term for "chest tube" is "thoracostomy[mh]". Searching this MeSH term retrieves articles manually reviewed by trained indexers who grouped all variant references to a chest tube (e.g., tube thoracostomy, chest tube, pigtail catheter) under this standardized term. Using MeSH terms helps retrieve all relevant records, regardless of how authors may have phrased the concept of interest in their manuscripts.

Wildcards Key concepts within the search should be linked to a MeSH term. However, when this is unavailable or impractical, wildcards—represented by the

Table 4.1 Examples of PubMed field tags to query specific metadata

	Field tag
Title	[ti]
Title/abstract	[tiab]
Language	[la]
Affiliation	[ad]
Text words	[tw]
MeSH terms	[mh]
Date of publication	[dp]
Author	[au]

asterisk—can capture spelling variations. For example, searching "hemothora*[ti]" would retrieve articles whose titles contain any word beginning with the stem *hemothora-*, including *hemothorax* (singular) and *hemothoraces* (plural).

Proximity search Standard searches may return irrelevant articles where keywords appear far apart throughout a manuscript. Proximity search—called using ":~N" within a field tag—increases precision by requiring specified words to appear within *N* words of each other.

For example, "chest tube hemothorax" [ti:~2] retrieves titles where the words "chest," "tube," and "hemothorax" appear within two words of each other. This search term would capture titles such as "Hemothorax requiring chest tube placement" but would not capture "tube thoracostomy for massive hemothorax" because the word "chest" is not in the title.

Boolean operators Boolean operators combine concepts logically. They must be capitalized.

AND retrieves articles that include all search terms. For example, "co-management AND surgery AND internal medicine" will retrieve articles where all three concepts appear somewhere in the article.

OR retrieves articles that include at least one of the search terms. For example, "Kidney stones OR kidney calculi OR renal calculi" will retrieve articles where any of the three terms appear in the article.

Last, *NOT* excludes articles that contain the search term. For example, "Skull base AND surgery NOT cadaver" will exclude articles that have the term "cadaver."

Parentheses can be used with Boolean operators to refine searches. For example, "Eating disorders AND teenagers OR adolescents" retrieves a different set of articles than "Eating disorders AND (teenagers OR adolescents)." The former is interpreted as "(Eating disorder AND teenagers) OR adolescents": this will retrieve articles related to eating disorders among teenagers, and any article mentioning adolescents in any context. The latter is aligned with the intended search for articles on eating disorders in the age group defined as teenagers or adolescents.

Familiarity with a search engine's logic allows you to retrieve the most relevant articles expeditiously. Rather than a generic search like "chest tube for hemothorax," a skilled researcher can construct a refined search, such as ("thoracic injuries/complications"[mh] OR "thoracic injuries/therapy"[mh] OR traumatic[tw] OR trauma[tiab] OR "thoracic injur*"[tw]) AND (hemothorax[mh] OR hemothora*) AND ("thoracostomy"[mh] OR thoracostom* OR "chest tub*" OR "chest tubes"[mh] OR drain*[tw]).

Avoiding the Cycle of Misinformation

Equally important as retrieving the right articles is ensuring they are cited accurately without misinterpretations. The article, "The Art of Writing a Scientific Article" by J Van de Geer et al., once accumulated hundreds of citations, even though it never existed. It was created by a publisher as an example of reference formatting, but was mistakenly cited by some researchers, prompting further citations by others who clearly never read this phantom article.

Many researchers do not read the articles they cite. Estimates suggest up to 20–25% of citations in biomedical literature are inaccurate misinterpretations, and our own research on the most highly cited articles in leading surgical journals found a 9% inaccurate citation rate. The practice of not reading articles is somewhat understandable: the volume of literature is overwhelming. Peer reviewers and editors do not have the time to fact-check every citation. Barring obvious false statements, they will assume authors will have done their due diligence. However, it is unclear how many principal investigators fact check every citation contributed by trainees or collaborators, and equally unclear how many trainees are taught about the magnitude of this problem.

A single inaccurate citation may seem harmless, but it can trigger a deadly spiral of misinformation propagation (Fig. 4.2).

Reviewers and editors assume the citation is accurate. Once the paper passes peer review, future authors cite the same "fact," trusting that earlier authors and reviewers verified it. The cycle continues until, over time, the inaccurate claim becomes repeatedly linked to the cited article. Eventually, the misinformation becomes entrenched as "well-established evidence" simply because it has been cited so many times, long after the original misinterpretation is forgotten.

Every author is responsible for every word in the manuscript, including all cited references. The onus is on every author to verify every fact cited, and to read the primary source, not just the title and abstract. Many non-experimental studies use declarative titles (e.g., "intervention *x* improves *y* outcome"), but on close review, there are many overstated or unsupported titles that pass peer review.

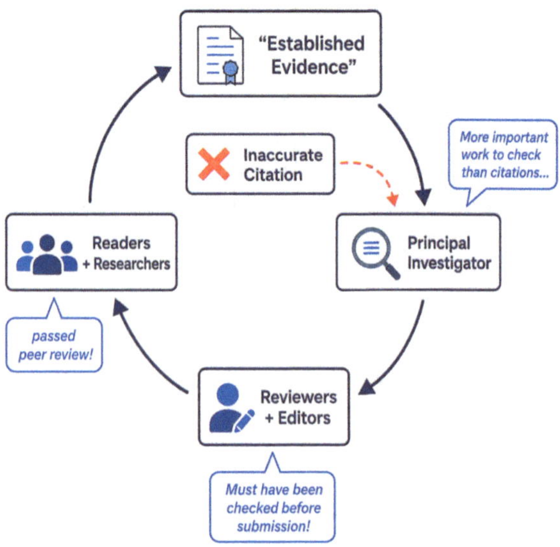

Fig. 4.2 The deadly spiral of misinformation propagation. An inaccurate citation can propagate unchecked when principal investigators, reviewers, and editors each assume that someone else has verified the source. After publication, the error may be further amplified by other authors who cite the work without independent fact-checking, until the misinformation accumulates enough citations to become entrenched as "evidence"

Fact-check every claim. Read the original article. Cite the primary source whenever possible, rather than the reference of a reference.

Reference Management Using Zotero

Most manuscripts undergo multiple revisions across several co-authors. During this process, it is common for citation superscripts to be deleted, misplaced, or not updated when text is reorganized. The result is a draft with missing or out-of-order references. Tracking down and linking the correct references is an unpleasant way to end a long project.

Using a reference manager is essential. It eliminates errors inherent to manual citation management and drastically improves efficiency, especially when resubmitting manuscripts to journals with different formatting requirements.

Several reference managers are available, including Zotero, EndNote, Mendeley, and Paperpile. The specific choice matters less than committing to *one* system and using it consistently across all projects. Master its features and apply them the same way, every time. Repetition fuels efficiency. This section highlights practical features of Zotero, a free and intuitive option that my team has relied on for years.

Web browser connectors Adding references to Zotero is straightforward using its web browser connectors, available for all major browsers. After navigating to a journal article or other citable webpage, clicking the Zotero connector automatically imports the citation into the selected library (described below). Zotero automatically downloads and attaches available article PDFs for full-text review. For citations imported without PDFs, full-text PDFs can be batch-retrieved using institutional journal subscriptions.

Libraries References can be organized into separate libraries for each project. The lead author can create a group library and invite team members. Any additions or edits sync automatically for everyone, ensuring the entire team is working from a single, consistent citation list. If working on multiple projects, users can specify the library each new citation should be imported into.

Microsoft Word and Google Docs plug-ins Zotero integrates directly with Microsoft Word and Google Docs. Once the plug-in is installed, citations can be inserted within the manuscript text with an "add citation button," which brings up a search bar to find any reference within your libraries. Zotero also generates a bibliography that updates automatically as citations are added or removed, or texts are rearranged. Each document can be formatted to match journal-specific citation styles, and Zotero includes over 10,000 citation styles. Selecting a new style will update all in-text citations and the bibliography with a single click.

Additional uses Beyond citation management, a Zotero library can store your own publications and streamline updates to your curriculum vitae. It can also serve as a reading library to store and annotate PDFs of articles and books, organized into folders. For example, you can maintain a shared folder of must-read articles for new lab members.

Mastering the research landscape requires understanding what is already known, identifying knowledge gaps, finding the relevant evidence thoroughly, and citing them responsibly. Amidst information overload, systematic reading habits, precise search strategies, and disciplined citation practices can ensure your study is built on integrity and does not spread misinformation.

Chapter 5
Why Most Studies Are False, and How Not to Conduct Most Studies

John Ioannidis' 2005 article "*Why Most Published Research Findings Are False*" forced an uncomfortable reckoning among researchers. Under relentless publish-or-perish pressure, studies are published with flawed designs, small samples, and avoidable biases, producing spurious findings that cannot be replicated. Twenty years later, whether the landscape is in a better state is unclear. Misinterpretations of foundational statistical concepts remain widespread, and recent enthusiasm for artificial intelligence has unleashed a wave of "AI studies" built on superficial methodological understanding.

This book is not a statistics or methodological textbook. However, a guide on academic publishing cannot ignore the uncomfortable reality that many published studies are unreliable. This book can teach the art of publishing efficiently. My hope, however, is that we use these tools to publish studies that matter—studies that advance knowledge, influence practice, and contribute meaningfully to advancing our fields.

This chapter highlights two cognitive traps and three methodological pitfalls that allow misinformation to seep into literature.

Trap # 1: Our Cognitive Shortcuts for Identifying "Good" Studies Are Flawed

With limited time and an overwhelming volume of literature, it is natural to rely on cognitive shortcuts to judge a study's quality (Fig. 5.1): randomized controlled trials versus observational studies; high versus low citation count; prestigious versus less prominent journal. When these cues look reassuring, we internalize a study's key finding and confidently pass it along as a citation or in conversation.

These shortcuts are misleading. Indeed, *well-designed* randomized controlled trials usually make a stronger case for causal inference, but adjudicating design quality

J. Choi, *The Research Publishing Playbook*,
https://doi.org/10.1007/978-3-032-28504-1_5

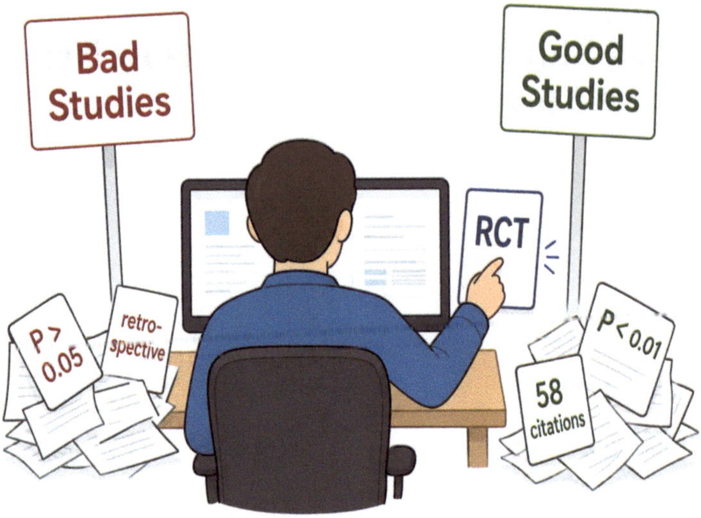

Fig. 5.1 Cognitive shortcuts to judge "good" vs "bad" studies. Facing limited time and information overload, we often rely on misleading signals to judge study quality

demands critical review rather than assumption. Even prominent randomized controlled trials have had their findings overturned (e.g., tight glucose control in the intensive care unit), and worse, revealed to be fraudulent. Citation counts are not reliable proxies for quality. They can reflect search engine visibility, keyword-rich titles, and the Matthew effect more than methodological rigor. High-impact journals often have stronger editorial processes, but no peer review pipeline is foolproof.

A habit of skepticism is essential. For hypothesis-driven studies, the null hypothesis should truly be the default expectation. The larger the claimed effect, the greater our skepticism should be. Skepticism will also be a safeguard for our own research; if we do not rigorously critique our own methods and assumptions, someone else will.

Trap # 2: Methodology Is Treated as an Afterthought

Many readers jump straight to the Results section: *What was the finding? What was the P value?* This inclination diverts attention from the most important part of a manuscript that determines whether results mean anything—the Methods. If the study design or analysis is flawed, the subsequent results and their interpretation are irrelevant (Fig. 5.2).

When we encounter complex or unfamiliar methods, we often assume this signals rigor. We may glance over the methods, trusting that peer reviewers with expertise would have vetted the details. Unfortunately, methodological expertise is rare, and many journals struggle to secure reviewers with the right training who can scrutinize methods in detail.

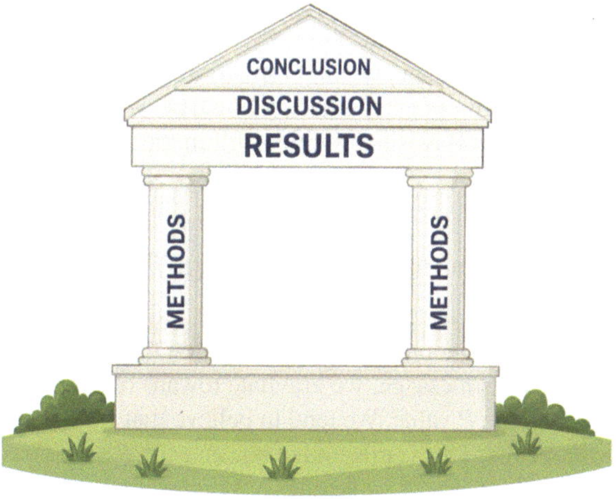

Fig. 5.2 The Methods form the foundation of every study. With flawed Methods, the Results, Discussion, and Conclusion are irrelevant

High-quality, reproducible science requires that every researcher takes responsibility for methodologic rigor. Every study should involve a methodologic expert from the beginning. Analyses should not begin until the methodologic blueprint has been finalized, just as no building construction begins before the architectural plan is complete. The belief that some studies are simple enough to "do my own statistics" can be dangerous. This problem is magnified in the era of large datasets and off-the-shelf, state-of-the-art algorithms, when it is easy to produce superficially impressive results. Reviewers, who assume that researchers would have done their methodologic due diligence, may mistakenly believe that these novel algorithms present pioneering research. Declarative titles can further inflate the perceived value of studies that lack methodological substance.

A study conducted without appropriate methodological expertise is like an operation performed by someone who never completed surgical training. Robust methodology is the cornerstone of every study; get it right from the beginning.

A comprehensive review of methodologic pitfalls across every discipline is impractical, but several prevalent errors deserve recognition by every researcher.

Pitfall 1: Confusing Bayesian Versus Frequentist Statistics

Human intuition is Bayesian. Most research is frequentist. Confusing the two—a Bayesian interpretation of frequentist results—is the culprit for many statistical misinterpretations.

For example, many researchers misinterpret 95% confidence intervals as a 95% probability that the true estimate lies within this interval. This is the correct interpretation for a Bayesian *credibility interval*. A frequentist 95% confidence interval is defined such that, across many hypothetical repetitions of the same study under the same assumptions, 95% of constructed intervals would contain the true estimate. The specific 95% confidence interval reported either does or does not contain the true estimate. If this definition is challenging to grasp, this is normal; frequentist statistics is not intuitive.

As another example, *P* values are commonly misinterpreted in the following manner: "$P = 0.02$ indicates a 98% probability that the observed effect is real." This is again a Bayesian-style interpretation. The frequentist *P* value says nothing about the probability of a hypothesis being true. Without a clear grasp of frequentist logic, our naturally Bayesian intuitions fill in the gaps, and misinterpretations proliferate.

Pitfall 2: Tying P *Values to Significance*

With limited memory capacity, we often seek a single takeaway from each study. In seeking this message, we gravitate toward one number to decide whether a finding matters: the *P* value. We tend to believe that smaller *P* values indicate more significant results. This is misguided because the *P*-value has little to do with *any* form of significance. The *P* value does not represent the probability of the result being true, the effect size, clinical relevance, or importance.

A *P* value represents the probability of seeing data that is as extreme or more extreme than what was observed, assuming the statistical model and all of its assumptions are correct. These assumptions range from the null hypothesis and sampling method to model specifications. Despite familiarity with the term, the *P* value is not intuitive, and its meaning is frequently misunderstood.

The conventional threshold of 0.05 is arbitrary. Why is 0.049 considered significant while 0.051 is not significant? Why do we speak of "*trending toward significance*"? Human cognition craves shortcuts to process information, and binary categorization reinforces the mistaken belief that *P* values reflect significance.

Additional errors surrounding *P* values are common. Using *P* values in baseline tables (often, Table 1) is misguided. *P* values imply hypothesis tests have been performed, yet most baseline tables are descriptive summaries, not inferential analyses. Declaring groups "balanced" because *P* values are >0.05 is incorrect, as is highlighting "statistically significant" baseline differences based on low *P* values. With large sample sizes, trivial differences will produce very small *P* values.

The fixation on *P* values has incentivized malicious practices such as p-hacking, wherein different models and study design specifications are employed until a "significant" finding results. What matters more than the actual *P* value is the underlying study design. No single number can substitute for a critical appraisal of the methods, which is the only way to judge whether a study's findings are credible.

Pitfall 3: Considering Multivariable Regression as Simple, Routine Analyses

Multivariable regression is ubiquitous, which misleads many researchers into treating it as routine analysis. It is not. Several common mistakes deserve discussion.

Confusing multivariate and multivariable "Multivariate" and "multivariable" regression are not interchangeable terms. The former refers to a model with multiple outcomes. Most researchers use multivariable models, which involve multiple predictors.

Confusing prediction and inference tasks These are distinct aims and require different study design considerations, from variable selection to exact statistical model choice. Inference aims to understand relationships between variables, while prediction concerns accurately forecasting outcomes.

Using the wrong regression model The regression model must match the type and distribution of the outcome. Standard logistic or linear regression models are often suboptimal for the task at hand. For example, hospital length of stay is typically right-skewed and is best modeled using a negative binomial regression or survival models rather than linear regression. Rare, rate-based count outcomes, such as the number of infections per N operations, are often better modeled using Poisson regression. Some variables that appear to be continuous are actually ordinal categorial variables—categories with a natural order, but unequal "spacing" between levels. These include Likert scales, pain scores, or the Injury Severity Score, and are often best modeled using ordinal logistic regression rather than linear regression. Hierarchical data, such as those concerning patients from multiple hospitals, should employ mixed-effects models.

Flawed variable selection Variable selection requires expert help. Including every variable from the baseline characteristics table or those with $P < 0.05$ on univariate analyses are two common flawed strategies. Variable selection is a complex topic that deserves a chapter of its own.

Assuming a variable is a confounder Not all non-outcome or non-exposure variables are confounders. Confounding describes a distinct relationship in the causal pathway between the exposure and the outcome. In inferential statistics, after all variables for a model are selected, their relationships must be mapped using a directed acyclic graph. These may include confounders, colliders, mediators, or effect modifiers. "Adjusting" for a variable that is not actually a confounder, as a confounder, can introduce biases, such as collider bias. Interpreting all coefficients resulting from a regression model the same way as that of the exposure is incorrect (i.e., Table 2 bias).

Most researchers are well-intentioned. However, several forces converge to create a perfect storm for false findings: cognitive shortcuts mislead us, methodological experts are insufficiently involved, and we overestimate our ability to perform "simple" analyses (Fig. 5.3).

There is no shortcut to high-quality research. Methodologic rigor should not be compromised, and experts must be involved in every study from the beginning.

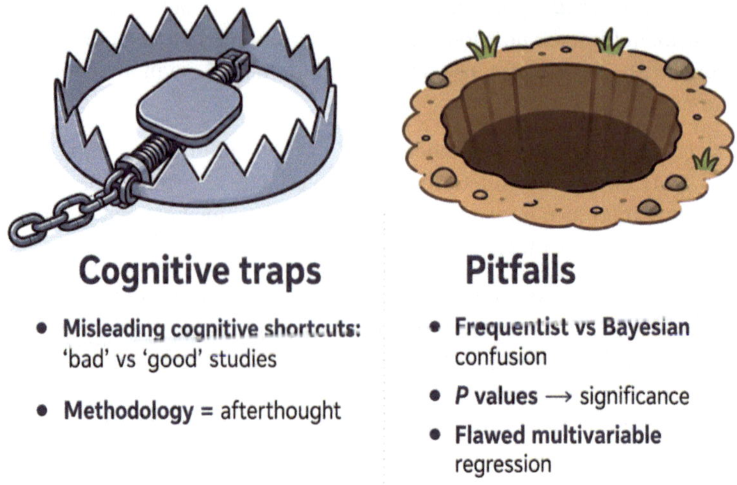

Fig. 5.3 Cognitive traps and methodologic pitfalls that threaten studies

Part II
The Writing

Chapter 6
Good Academic Writing Is Not "Academic Writing"

Academic writing is often associated with jargon, dense writing, and convoluted prose. In reality, good academic writing is just good writing: clear, direct, and effective in communicating a message. The "academic" piece only refers to the topic and target audience.

Recall that editors and peer reviewers volunteer their time. A well-written manuscript will allow them to focus on what really matters: the quality of research. Even a well-conducted study, if presented in poor writing, will irritate readers. If reviewers have to reread sentences to understand what is being communicated, annoyance will seep into their judgment of the science.

An unfortunate reality is that most manuscripts will not be read by many readers once published. Many will cite articles based on the abstract or title alone. However, for those that do attract readers to its full text, a poorly-written manuscript will lose readers immediately. Writing well may not be a forté for many academics but is just as important as conducting good research and must be practiced deliberately.

This chapter presents practical strategies to improve writing quality and includes examples to illustrate how writing can be effectively revised.

Practical Strategies to Improve Writing

Read the manuscript out loud Reading out loud helps highlight awkward phrasing, unclear logic, and long sentences. *If something sounds "off," this needs to be rewritten.* A sentence that requires more than a typical breath to read is typically too long and will lose readers. Clear writing should sound right.

Every sentence should flow logically If a sentence has to be reread because it does not make sense, the logic is likely flawed. Every sentence should make logical

J. Choi, *The Research Publishing Playbook*,
https://doi.org/10.1007/978-3-032-28504-1_6

sense. Word choice should be precise. Active voice, rather than passive voice, is clearer. Double negatives are challenging to follow.

Avoid acronyms Acronyms are commonly employed to reduce word counts. However, unless the acronym is universally familiar to the target audience (e.g., "CT scans" for physicians), it can force readers to pause to recall its meaning. Newly coined acronyms may be familiar to researchers but will be disruptive to readers. Unless universally recognized or essential (e.g., marketing a new treatment using its acronym), avoid acronyms. If acronyms are employed, they should be spelled out the first time they appear.

Do not confuse e.g. and i.e. "E.g." and "i.e." are not interchangeable. "E.g.," the Latin abbreviation for *exempli gratia*, means "for example" and should precede a list of examples. "I.e.," the Latin abbreviation for id est, means "that is" and should be used to clarify a preceding statement. For example, "fruits (e.g., strawberries, blueberries) are delicious."

Use consistent terminology Manuscripts often discuss several key concepts continuously. These concepts should be described using consistent terminology. For example, a manuscript discussing "artificial intelligence algorithms" should use the term "artificial intelligence algorithm" consistently, rather than using multiple terms such as "artificial intelligence tools," "artificial intelligence models," or "machine learning models." A "patients with 90-day readmissions" cohort should not be described using heterogeneous terms such as "readmitted patients," "patients readmitted within 90 days," or "the readmitted group."

Consistency prevents reader confusion. It is critical to remember that readers will not be familiar with concepts you may have spent months indulged in.

Minimize adjectives and adverbs Adjectives and adverbs often add little and create clutter. If a sentence works without an adjective or adverb, delete them.

Use the fewest possible words Word limits are caps, not targets to reach. Communicate your research to readers using the fewest possible words. Brevity enforces clarity. Every paragraph should have a single purpose; every sentence should serve that purpose; and every word must be essential.

After completing a full draft, read the manuscript out loud and at the end of every sentence, ask—is this sentence essential? If not, it should be removed. See if multiple sentences can be combined into a single shorter sentence. Delete adjectives and adverbs. Punctuations such as semi-colons (;), colons (:), and em-dashes (—), and writing in the active voice can often eliminate several words. A concise, clear manuscript where every word is purposeful will be appreciated by readers. Concise writing is good writing.

Use the supplement If the journal allows, delegate dense methodological descriptions and nonessential results to the Supplement. This allows communicating essential messages in the main manuscript body, while interested readers can review details. For example, if sensitivity analyses yielded similar findings as the primary analysis, a simple statement and reference to the Supplement can suffice.

Do not regurgitate tables and figures Use tables and figures effectively to make your manuscript less dense. Do not restate every table cell in writing; this adds unnecessary noise. Let tables and figures speak for themselves, and reserve the text only for essential emphases.

Overcoming Writer's Block

Writer's block is common. An effective way to overcome it is simple: just keep writing. Rather than trying to perfect a sentence or find the best word, just get the words down on paper. Writing a series of perfect sentences is less efficient than multiple passes of writing revisions. Each pass can focus on specific ways to improve the manuscript. One pass can fill logic gaps. Another can focus on brevity. Another can refine the tone and style.

Like any skill, writing improves with practice. Even if for a couple of minutes, writing consistently every day and reading good writing will help. Strunk and White's *The Elements of Style* is a fantastic book for anyone aiming to improve their writing.

Example Texts

We will illustrate several examples to highlight common ways writing can be revised for clarity, precision, and brevity.

Example 1 An Excerpt from a Hypothetical Introduction
Original: *Undergraduate students often report that research productivity is an important metric for medical school application competitiveness. Many believe that their chances of admission will be higher the more they are involved with research. Research productivity including presenting abstracts at conferences, and publishing peer-reviewed manuscripts is consistently higher for admitted applicants compared to non-admitted applicants suggesting its importance for application competitiveness among undergrads.*

Example of improvement opportunities:

Inconsistent terminology:

- Undergraduate students vs applicants vs undergrads

Nonessential sentence and phrase:

- The second sentence is redundant.
- "Suggesting its importance for application competitiveness ...": the same fact has been communicated for the third time.

Clutter:

- "Presenting abstracts at conferences" → conference presentations
- "Publishing peer-reviewed manuscripts" → publications

Revised: *For applicants, research productivity is an important differentiator in medical school admissions; accepted applicants have more conference presentations and publications than those who are not accepted.*

Example 2 Hypothetical Excerpt from Results in an Observational Study
Original: *Patients who underwent an operation were more likely to be male (32%* vs *22%; P < 0.02), older (32(30–36)* vs *46(40–49), P < 0.045), white, (42%* vs *34%, P < 0.001), Asian (15%* vs *12%, P < 0.001), African American (23%* vs *20%, P < 0.001), hospitalized longer (5(7–9)* vs *3(2–4) days, P < 0.001), on aspirin (12%* vs *6%, P < 0.02), experience ICU stay (3%* vs *1.2%, P < 0.043) and die (0.5%* vs *0.1%, P < 0.03; Table 1).*

Example of improvement opportunities:
Imprecise language:

- The sentence does not specify the comparator group.
- "More likely" suggests likelihood was evaluated. Likelihood is a specific statistical terminology. The authors mean to say, "a higher proportion of."
- What authors mean by "die" is unclear; everyone dies at some point. The definition may have been specified in the methods (e.g., inpatient mortality, 30-day mortality), but consistent terminology should be used.
- The authors likely conducted chi-square or Fisher's exact test to compare the distribution of race categories (white, Asian, African American, etc.) between the two groups, which yielded one *P*-value across all groups. These tests evaluate differences across the overall distribution of categories, not between specific categories.

Redundancy with Table 1:

- Table 1 typically illustrates baseline differences between two groups. Hypothesis testing, and therefore *P*-values, is unnecessary in a descriptive table. It is unclear what meaningful message is being communicated by rewriting data that is already summarized in a table.

Revised: *Table 1 illustrates differences in baseline characteristics between patients who did and did not undergo an operation.*

Example 3 Hypothetical First Paragraph of Introduction
Original: Clinical prediction models (CPMs) support physicians in clinical decision-making with the aim of improving patient outcomes. CPMs aim to provide

diagnostic or prognostic analyses based on large quantities of data while mitigating human bias, fatigue, and error. Supplementing a physician's expertise gained through years of extensive training and patient-facing clinical care with CPMs offers a novel two-pronged approach to facilitate improved clinical decision-making. Understandably, there has been a surge in the volume of literature proposing original prediction models. There remains, however, concern that this fruitful production of CPMs has yet to make a substantial impact on clinical practice. Successful advancement along the pathway from database to bedside is challenging as this demands transparent development, independent validation, staged implementation, and trust and acceptance among stakeholders.

Example of improvement opportunities:

Lack of meaningful focus:

- Every paragraph in a manuscript should serve a clear purpose. For example, the first paragraph of an Introduction should draw readers in and establish why the study matters. The example paragraph opens with a generic definition, one that the target audience likely knows. The first three sentences are redundant and do not advance the narrative.
- It is only by the fifth sentence that readers get a hint of the problem the study may be addressing. However, the magnitude of the problem is unclear—what do the authors mean by a "surge in the volume of literature"? No data is presented to support the concern that "fruitful production of CPMs has yet to make a substantial impact on clinical practice."
- After suggesting there is a concern regarding CPM's, the final sentence appears to weaken the problem by offering reasons why translation is difficult. This decreases the sense of scale or urgency that this paragraph should be advancing. By the end of the paragraph, readers have learned little beyond a general sense that there is a surge in CPM papers and these have yet to make a substantial impact on clinical practice.

Unnecessary acronym:

- "CPM" is not a universally recognized acronym. In the above section, did you have to pause, even briefly, to recall that "CPM" referred to clinical prediction models? That momentary interruption is exactly the problem. Unless an acronym is universally recognized or essential to the manuscript's goal, it should be avoided.

Revised: Despite methodological advances and growing interest, most clinical prediction models remain confined to research publications. Nearly 30,000 model development studies have been published between 2010 and 2015, yet fewer than 10% have undergone any external validation, and fewer than 1% have demonstrated real-world clinical use [citations]. The striking imbalance between model development and subsequent evaluation highlights a central problem: a systemic failure to translate models from database to bedside.

Chapter 7
Title, Abstract, Introduction: Lights, Camera, Action!

Recall that the optimal research workflow is a parallel process wherein manuscript writing and other research activities can occur simultaneously. Especially for team-based projects, there is no need to write the manuscript in the order in which it ultimately appears. Team members familiar with the methodology should draft the *Methodology* and *Limitations* sections before experiments begin. Most limitations are methodologic. At the same time, others can draft the *Introduction* and parts of the *Discussion* section that don't require knowing the results.

Writing in parallel improves efficiency and guards against a common pitfall: the progressive decline in writing quality throughout a manuscript. When writing is deferred until analyses are complete, teams are worn out, and writing can be perceived as a final hurdle rather than an integral part of the scientific process. As a result, early sections of a manuscript undergo extensive revisions, while later sections—often the most intellectually demanding—are written in haste (Fig. 7.1).

This book presents chapters in typical manuscript order for familiarity. However, in practice, manuscript sections should rarely be written sequentially.

The Title: Intentional Versus Incidental Audience

The title is the most widely read part of any manuscript. A well-crafted title can attract the audience's attention and increase the likelihood that your work reaches people who can carry your ideas forward and advance the field. The title is your manuscript's handshake with the world and must consider two distinct audiences: the intentional and the incidental.

The ***intentional audience*** refers to those actively searching for information related to your manuscript's topic. These may be clinicians seeking guidance for patient care, researchers conducting literature reviews, or teams assembling a

J. Choi, *The Research Publishing Playbook*,
https://doi.org/10.1007/978-3-032-28504-1_7

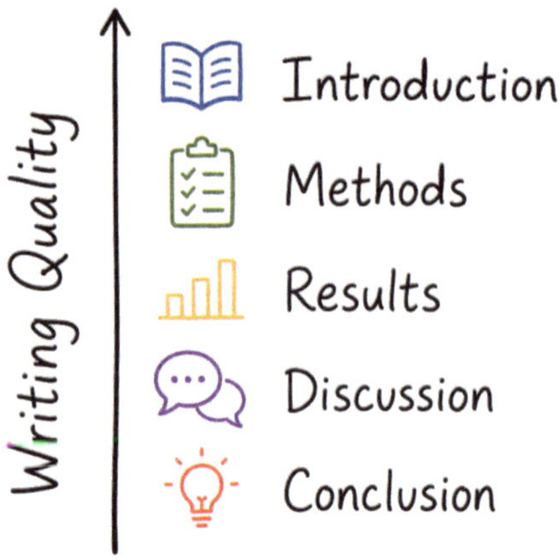

Fig. 7.1 Progressive decline in writing quality. Manuscripts written sequentially after experiments finish often exhibit a gradual decline in writing quality across sections

systematic review. Most will search online through general search engines or academic databases, and most will not scroll beyond the first page of results.

Search engines and databases use proprietary algorithms, but keyword relevance is a major driver. Ask:

Who do I want this manuscript to reach?
If I were them, what search terms would I use?

Titles that closely match expected search queries rank higher and are more likely to be read. Try this exercise: search any topic of interest. The top results often include manuscripts whose titles match your query exactly, and these papers tend to have high citation counts. Once citation counts rise, high user engagement boosts its priority in search results: "the rich get richer."

It may be tempting to attract attention using clever titles with rhymes, wordplay, or acronyms. However, if your title doesn't appear on the first page of results, creativity does not matter—readers will never see it.

The ***incidental audience*** refers to those who come across your title by chance—on social media, conference slides, or a journal's table of contents. These are window shoppers: they were not searching for your work but may stop to read further if the title compels attention.

Attempts to compel this group's attention often lead authors to craft titles that overstate findings, framing results as definitive, implying causality, or making sweeping claims the study was not designed to prove. This misleading practice is especially dangerous in a landscape where many researchers cite studies without reading beyond the title. Misleading titles can seed misinformation that circulates unchecked until they become entrenched as facts.

Unless the study was designed to establish causality beyond reasonable doubt (e.g., a well-designed randomized controlled trial), a title should not make a declarative statement.

The Effective Title

If flashy or declarative titles are discouraged, what is an effective title? Excluding manuscripts published in highly visible, broadly read journals, the *intentional* audience will usually outnumber the *incidental*. The title should be crafted to maximize discoverability for the intentional audience by incorporating strategic keywords tied to your study's core elements.

Consider a basic science study on the mechanism of a protein involved in appendicitis. If the protein is involved in other pathologies, the title could reflect this broader relevance and increase discoverability by researchers in those areas. Similarly, if the study employed an innovative methodology applicable beyond protein modeling, highlighting this in the title could draw interest from a broader audience.

For instance, instead of "*The Role of Protein X in Appendicitis,*" more effective titles may be:

"Proteomics and Surgery: the Role of Protein X in Appendicitis"
"The Role of Protein X in Appendicitis: Leveraging [methodology] to Characterize [mechanism]"

These titles incorporate keywords that broaden discoverability of the study's reach without misrepresenting its scope.

Manuscripts concerning niche topics often have limited appeal to the *incidental* audience. You may consider two strategies:

1. Targeting a broad journal with a higher impact factor and larger total readership
2. Targeting a specialized journal where the total readership is smaller, but a higher proportion is actively engaged with your topic.

A journal with a higher impact factor does not necessarily increase the likelihood of greater interest in or citations for *your* paper. The impact factor represents the total number of citations divided by the number of citable articles in a journal over a two-year period. The metric summarizes a non-normal distribution of citations across many studies, and may be skewed by a few highly cited review articles or popular topics unrelated to yours.

Submitting to a specialized journal, despite a lower impact factor, can be the more strategic choice. While the total readership may be smaller, it may include a more active research community with an interest in your topic, which may translate into more meaningful engagement and citations over time.

The Abstract

Alongside the title, the abstract is the most widely read part of a manuscript. For manuscripts behind a paywall, it may be the only part many readers can access. The abstract must accomplish two tasks:

1. Convince readers that the full text is worth reading.
2. Deliver the manuscript's key message with convincing authority.

In general, the abstract should be written last. After the manuscript is finalized, the most important elements should be distilled and presented front and center. Trimming down from a polished manuscript ensures the most widely read part of the manuscript is truly a "crème de la crème" summary.

Readers will not remember every detail the manuscripts they read. Years or even weeks later, they will recall a single key message. The abstract's purpose is to embed this key message and outline its validity by highlighting the knowledge gap addressed, robust methods employed, and compelling results. Every word in the abstract must serve this ultimate purpose.

Most journals require structured abstracts (typically 100–300 words) with four sections. Below are suggestions for each section:

The introduction/objective. Highlight a critical and urgent knowledge gap. State the aim concisely. Eliminate background information not directly related to the aim and generic statements.

Methods/results. A study may involve many analyses, such as subgroup and sensitivity analyses. Only include methods and results that are essential to the key message. Highlight study population characteristics for readers to gauge external validity, methods that signal rigor, and the primary findings.

Conclusion. Deliver the one-sentence takeaway. If space permits, state the implications of the takeaway.

Before submission, review abstracts from target journals to become familiar with winning strategies.

The Introduction

The Introduction can and should be drafted before any data collection or analysis begins. Andrew Ibrahim and Justin Dimick's Chapter, "*Writing for Impact*" outlines a powerful framework for writing an impactful introduction, which this section will build on. The effective introduction achieves three goals using three paragraphs: highlight the importance of a problem; highlight a knowledge gap; and state the study aim and hypothesis. For shorter manuscripts, the second and third goals could be combined into one paragraph.

Importance of a problem The introduction should speak to both domain experts and non-experts. Domain experts already know the relevance of a problem. Non-experts often have a specific reason they are reading the manuscript beyond the abstract. Long, textbook background tours are unnecessary and unhelpful for readers. Rather than a generic fact, a direct problem statement can be a captivating first sentence. Use a few targeted sentences to convey the magnitude and importance of the problem.

Some authors struggle because they try to highlight their study's importance to too broad an audience. Remember, the lay public is not the target audience for most research manuscripts, and the introduction's purpose is not to convince *everyone* of the study's importance—only your intended audience.

Knowledge gap Other groups have likely attempted to answer the same or similar problems. Why is it that you decided to put a research team together and dedicate time to this study? The typical motivation is to answer an unanswered question: to fill a knowledge gap. It is critical to state this knowledge gap and highlight why filling this gap matters. Who will benefit from the answer? Why does this question need an answer now? Even if your study won't definitively solve a problem or change the field overnight, this paragraph must outline the next step your study enables.

Study aim/hypothesis The third paragraph can often be written using three sentences. The first sentence should state the study aim ("We aimed to..."). For hypothesis-driven research, the last sentence should state the hypothesis ("We hypothesized..."). In between, the second sentence can preview key methodological strengths that signal credibility, such as using a contemporary database or novel technique.

A consistent writing template can reduce decision fatigue and accelerate the writing process as experience accumulates. Solidify your writing formula as much as possible. For many manuscripts, you should be able to predict the purpose of the *N*th sentence of the *N*th paragraph.

There are many studies that could be cited to highlight the importance of a problem or a knowledge gap: what belongs in the *Introduction*, rather than the *Discussion*? As will be detailed in a later chapter, a part of the Discussion includes summarizing existing literature. Recall that every paragraph in a manuscript serves a specific purpose, and that the fewest possible words should be used to achieve that purpose. Studies that are essential for highlighting the importance of a problem or a knowledge gap should be included in the Introduction. These studies can be introduced to the extent of achieving the *Introduction's* purpose, and be detailed more in depth later in the *Discussion*.

Pitfalls

We conclude this chapter with three pitfalls that undermine effective Introductions.

1. **Wordiness**. The introduction is a gateway, not the destination. More words create more opportunities for confusion. Use the fewest words to logically guide the reader toward your goal: outline a problem's importance, highlight a knowledge gap, and state your study aim and hypothesis.
2. **Claims of being "first."** Be cautious saying "this study is first to." If a reviewer can refute this claim, they will, and the reset of your manuscript's credibility will

be damaged. Avoid claiming priority unless this is essential. If you must, make sure to conduct a thorough review of the literature to support this claim and qualify your statement with "to our knowledge."

3. **Logic leaps**. Two common forces produce illogical leaps that confuse readers. The first is *researcher familiarity bias*. After months immersed in a study, the motivation for the study and the importance of everything that was done feel self-evident. Connections that seem too obvious to state often go unstated. However, your readers do not share this familiarity. They need step-by-step logic to follow the manuscript.

   Second, many teams defer manuscript writing to the end. By then, authors are often too fatigued to catch subtle logical gaps. Additionally, authors may unintentionally reshape the narrative to better align with their findings. This post hoc reframing can create a noticeable disconnect between the study aim and actual narrative. Writing the introduction before conducting analyses or seeing any results ensures the writing reflects the true, unbiased purpose of the study.

Chapter 8
Methods: The Bedrock of Every Study

Methodology is the bedrock of every study. Reviewers could reasonably reject a manuscript based on the Methods alone if the study was fundamentally incapable of answering its stated aim. Noble motivations or interesting findings are irrelevant if the methodology is weak. The Methods deserves the greatest share of planning, the most rigorous editing, and the most vigilant critical review.

Involve a Methodologic Expert

Research begins with the Methods: the Methods should be the first section of a manuscript that is written. This point was presented in previous chapters, but warrants repetition: every study must involve a methodologic expert from the beginning.

The stakes of a research study are high. Findings can advance a field, improve lives, or improve our understanding of the world. On the other hand, if flawed, it wastes the time of the research team and readers, spreads misinformation, and undermines public trust. Once published, our names are permanently linked to a manuscript, even if the study is later retracted. It is in every research team's interest to ensure their study is grounded in rigorous methodology.

Think of research as an operation. If a loved one were to undergo an operation, you would want more than someone who understands basic principles of operating. You would want a surgeon with formal training, experience performing that specific operation, who understands the nuances of performing the operation safely, mitigating complications, and optimizing the potential for the best recovery. The same principles apply to your methodologic expert. Do not seek a "statistician." "Statistics" is an enormous field. Most statisticians may have a general understanding of many methodologies to make recommendations, but your study needs someone who has direct experience with the required methodology and understands its

J. Choi, *The Research Publishing Playbook*,
https://doi.org/10.1007/978-3-032-28504-1_8

nuances and pitfalls. As soon as a study is conceived, the principal investigator's first job should be to identify this expert.

A methodologic expert is also invaluable for writing the Methods effectively. Many reviewers or readers may not be familiar with the employed methodology. Those who understand the techniques most deeply are best equipped to explain complex designs clearly and concisely.

Follow Appropriate Reporting Guidelines

Several organizations have developed reporting guidelines to improve research quality, reproducibility, and transparency. These guidelines contain elements relevant not only to the Methods but also to the entire manuscript. For example, the EQUATOR network (equator-network.org) houses reporting guidelines for most study designs encountered in health research, including:

CONSORT—randomized control trials
STROBE—observational studies
PRISMA—systematic reviews
TRIPOD—clinical decision support tools
CHEERS—economic evaluations
SQUIRE—quality improvement studies

The National Institutes of Health also maintains a similar compendium (https://www.nlm.nih.gov/services/research_report_guide.html), including MIAME (microarray experiments), REMARK (tumor marker studies), and COREQ (interviews and focus groups).

As an example, the Table 8.1 presents a subsection of the STROBE checklist for cross-sectional studies.

For statistical methods, the guideline not only recommends reporting well-known elements, such as controlling for confounding, but also less-frequently reported elements, such as testing for interactions, addressing missing data, and

Table 8.1 A portion of the Methods section within the STROBE checklist for cross-sectional studies

Bias	Describe any efforts to address potential sources of bias
Study size	Explain how the study size was arrived at
Quantitative variables	Explain how quantitative variables were handled in the analyses. If applicable, describe which groupings were chosen and why
Statistical methods	(*a*) Describe all statistical methods, including those used to control for confounding
	(*b*) Describe any methods used to examine subgroups and interactions
	(*c*) Explain how missing data were addressed
	(*d*) If applicable, describe analytical methods taking account of sampling strategy
	(*e*) Describe any sensitivity analyses

sensitivity analysis. Reviewing these guidelines often reveals essential study design elements that warrant expert methodologist guidance before data collection or analysis begins.

The Methods should explicitly state adherence to the appropriate guideline, and the checklist should be submitted as a Supplement. This signals rigor to reviewers immediately.

Use Subheadings

The Methods is the blueprint that outlines exactly how a study was performed and how results were derived. For many readers, this is the densest section that is most cumbersome to read. Recall the **researcher familiarity bias**: complex analyses and nuanced study design decisions are well-known to the research team, who may be unaware of the exclusivity of this knowledge. Reviewers and readers are not privy to the many lab meetings and months of discussions that shaped the study. To understand why a study was designed in a particular manner or how results were derived, they rely entirely on the Methods section.

Structured subheadings aligned with each sequence of planning and executing the study can guide readers through the Methods logically. For example, the typical sequence for health services research studies is outlined below:

IRB and Reporting Guideline Researchers begin by seeking an institutional review board approval or waiver, then refer to the appropriate reporting guideline (e.g., STROBE). The first two sentences of the methods might read:

> We obtained institutional review board approval from [IRB name, protocol number] and followed the [name of reporting guideline] (Supplement).

Data source Next, researchers define the study population and select a data source. Provide a brief description of the data source (e.g., institutional registry, administrative dataset) and the reason for selecting this particular source. This context allows readers to evaluate (1) whether the source is appropriate to answer the study aim and (2) the study's external validity. For example, if a clinical study only included subjects from high-volume academic hospitals, the findings may not generalize to patients in rural community hospitals.

Inclusion and Exclusion Criteria After identifying the data source, researchers use inclusion and exclusion criteria to select their study population. Inclusion criteria specify eligibility characteristics (e.g., age, setting), while exclusion criteria describe disqualifying characteristics. Unless the rationale is self-devident, reasons for exclusion should be stated explicitly. Remember, readers only know what is written.

Sample size calculation Some studies warrant sample size calculations. Sample size calculation techniques are beyond this book's scope, but with expert guidance, the employed technique, assumptions, and supporting references should be outlined.

Primary and secondary outcomes By this point, readers may be several hundred words into the manuscript. It is not uncommon to finish reading a dense Methods section, only to forget the study aim, and have to re-read the Methods again. Present the primary and secondary outcomes early so readers can recall the study aim and whether the design logically addressed the stated aim.

Why a specific outcome was chosen may need clarification. For example, if the primary outcome was 30-day mortality, why was this chosen over 60-day or 90-day mortality? If a specific quality of life measurement tool was used, why was the particular tool chosen among many others? If applicable, strategies to capture the outcome such as follow-up protocols should be detailed.

Variables Most studies involve capturing many variables relevant to the analysis. These variables may help characterize the study population or may be candidate covariates for statistical modeling. Listing all captured variables in a long paragraph is often unhelpful. Consider this sentence:

> From the database, we extracted patients' age, sex, ZIP code, health insurance status, race/ethnicity, hospital length of stay, inpatient mortality, intensive care unit length of stay, complications including…

Readers will not enjoy reading a laundry list of variables within an already-dense Methods section. Instead, highlight those that require clarification (e.g., how post-operative complication was defined in the database) or are integral to the subsequent analysis, and relegate the rest to a supplement.

Missing data If applicable, include strategies for handling missing data as a separate section. Explicitly describe assumptions regarding the missing data type and your strategy (e.g., multiple imputations).

Analysis The analysis section is typically the most dense. Describe analyses in the logical order in which experiments were performed. Justify major decisions, such as why a particular statistical model was chosen, why particular variables were included or excluded, and how sensitivity analyses evaluated various assumptions. If the study includes a complex series of analyses, a Figure that provides a broad overview of analytic steps and how they relate can provide an overarching perspective for readers (Fig. 8.1).

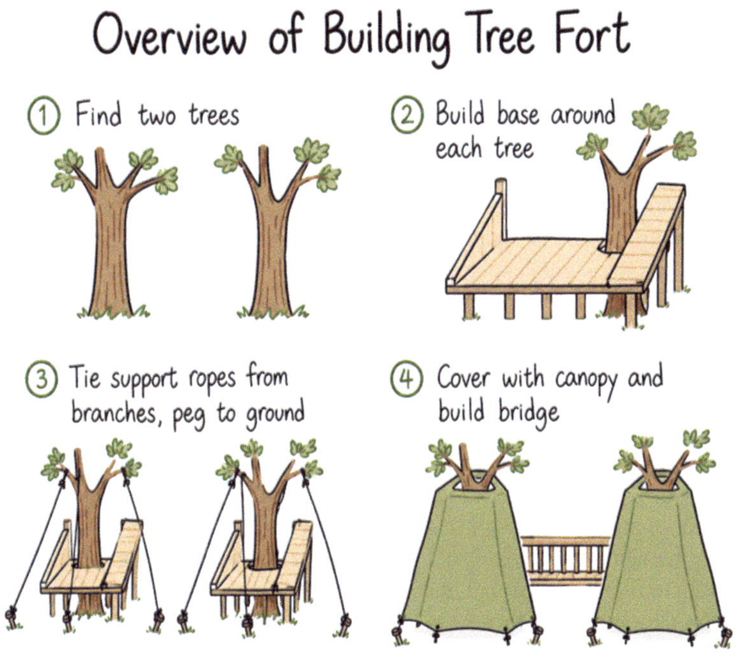
Overview of Building Tree Fort
① Find two trees
② Build base around each tree
③ Tie support ropes from branches, peg to ground
④ Cover with canopy and build bridge

Fig. 8.1 Methodologic overview of complex analyses. A high-level schematic illustrating how individual analytic steps relate to one another (in this example, steps of building a tree fort) can orient readers while they work through the details of each analysis

Consider Supplemental Files

What details should be included in the Methods? Ideally, enough information for interested readers to fully replicate the study. A Supplemental Methods section can keep main Methods concise while providing complete technical details for interested readers.

For example, the main Methods can highlight key analytic decisions and steps, while material that may overwhelm general readers can be relegated to the Supplemental Methods. Many journals impose word limits on the main text, but have no such restrictions on supplemental files.

Consider sharing the analytic code publicly (e.g., via Github). Sharing the code facilitates reproducibility and allows others to adapt your approach and build upon your research.

Pitfalls

Three pitfalls can undermine writing effective Methods.

1. **Not knowing the audience**. Calibrate the language and detail to your audience. For example, a study that employed advanced machine learning techniques may need a variable depth of technical description depending on the target audience (e.g., computer science journal or a general biomedical journal). Complex language does not signal expertise; clarity does.
2. **Losing sight of the forest for the trees**. Meandering descriptions or excessive details can obscure the readers' main purpose for reading the Methods: evaluating whether the study was designed and analyzed to answer the stated aim. Longer Methods do not necessarily translate to better replicability or transparency. Concise writing, subheadings, and supplemental files are your allies.
3. **Including Results in the Methods**. Numbers and findings produced by analyses belong in Results, not Methods. For example, a flow diagram that outlines the number of subjects through stages of the study belongs in the Results. However, fixed characteristics of a data source belong in Methods. For example, that an administrative database includes data from *N* number of states provides context for readers; this statistic belongs in the Methods.

Chapter 9
Results: The Words-Figures-Tables Monopoly

Months or years of work lead to this section. Your team set out to answer a question, designed a study, and executed the analysis. The Results is where you present what the study found. Conventions for presenting Results vary across disciplines, but all readers will have two questions:

What was the finding?
Do the presented facts support that finding?

This chapter outlines fundamental principles and strategies to ensure your Results are factual and worthy of readers' trust.

Resist the Temptation to Overstate Findings

It is natural for researchers to want meaningful results. From the principal investigator to trainees, everyone invests substantial time into a project and develops a deep desire to produce influential findings and to know that their efforts mattered. This desire creates a temptation to portray results as more definitive or noteworthy than they are. This temptation must be fiercely resisted.

Practices such as manipulating data and "p-hacking" are not only unethical but are career-ending. Prominent researchers have experienced very public downfalls; a career built on scientific misconduct will fall. Even without overt misconduct, overstating or overinterpreting results erodes credibility. Many feel discouraged when findings do not reach "statistical significance," leading to the flawed belief that "negative" studies—a misnomer—lack value. This is incorrect. If a study was designed rigorously and analyzed appropriately, the findings are valuable, regardless of alignment with the hypothesis. Meaningful study aims investigated rigorously deserve accurate reporting.

J. Choi, *The Research Publishing Playbook*,
https://doi.org/10.1007/978-3-032-28504-1_9

The Results should be strictly factual. The Discussion offers ample space for interpretation. The goal of the Results is to clearly present findings in a logical manner, not to persuade. Well-written Results will allow readers to infer meaning from presented facts.

Mirror the Methods

The Methods section outlined the study design and analytic plan in a logical sequence. Results should be presented in this same sequence. If these two sections were printed and laid side-by-side, they should align like the rungs of a ladder (Fig. 9.1).

Most Methods begin with the data source, inclusion and exclusion criteria, and resulting study population. Most Results should begin by describing this study population, and how they were derived using a flow diagram (e.g., CONSORT flow diagram).

If multiple analyses were performed, present findings in the order in which they were described in the Methods. A logical series of findings will align well with a logical sequence of experiments. As in the Methods section, use subheadings to orient readers and offer visual milestones.

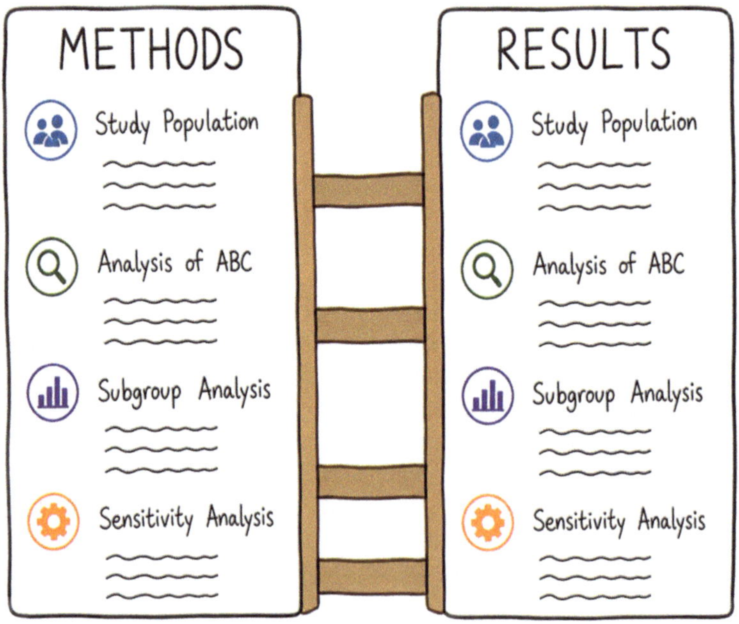

Fig. 9.1 Alignment of Methods and Results. Content in the Methods and Results should correspond directly and be presented in the same sequential order. This structural consistency improves clarity and readability for readers

Use the Fewest Possible Words

The fewest possible words should be used to communicate findings effectively. Readers will rarely retain more than one key message from a manuscript. Present a logical series of facts that lead readers to this message. Every word should serve this purpose.

Words are often less efficient than figures or tables. Consider the pages of a manuscript as prime real estate. Fill the space using the combination of words, figures, or tables that requires the least space and falls within journal guidelines. There is rarely a need to restate information in multiple formats. For example, repeating every cell of a baseline demographics table in text is unhelpful. Instead, highlight facts that serve a specific purpose, such as characteristics that influence external validity.

Secondary analyses or detailed findings do not always belong in the main text. For example, if sensitivity analyses corroborate the primary analysis, a simple sentence such as "Sensitivity analyses found similar estimates (Supplement figure x)" is sufficient.

Design Effective Figures and Tables

Effective figures and tables should be designed as stand-alone units. If they were cropped and shown on a presentation slide without the manuscript title, readers should be able to understand their purpose.

Titles should be succinct and precise. The first table in many biomedical studies describes baseline characteristics. "Baseline characteristics" is vague. "*Baseline characteristics of US adults undergoing operative or non-operative management of appendicitis*" is a meaningful stand-alone title.

Use figures and tables only when they add value. For example, a two-row table describing basic outcomes may be more efficiently presented using one-sentence text. Because tables and figures are often provided as separate files and are not in line with text, unnecessary items that disrupt the reading process can be frustrating. That a journal allows up to five tables of figures does not mean all must be used.

Figures

Figures should never be unedited exports from Excel, R, or Python. Raw outputs are obvious and appear unprofessional. Several considerations are worth mentioning:

Color schemes If colors are used to distinguish groups or effect sizes, use palettes tested for individuals with color vision deficiencies. For example, red-green and blue-yellow schemes should be avoided. Color schemes should be standardized across figures in a manuscript. For example, consistent colors should be used to indicate higher and lower values, or to identify specific subgroups.

Text and typography All text, axis labels, and tick marks within figures must be legible without zooming. Formatting and alignment must be intentional (e.g., bold, centered). Typeface (e.g., Arial, Helvetica) should be standardized across all figures. If you find text formatting using statistical software challenging, import the image into a more familiar program, such as Microsoft PowerPoint, to adjust text manually.

Legends All symbols, shapes, and scales should be interpretable. For example, small circles and squares may be indistinguishable. Heatmap gradients should use a numerical scale and color scheme appropriate for the data (e.g., log-transformed values). Legends should be large enough to read without magnification.

Resolution Do not use screenshots or low-resolution images. Figures should remain crisp when displayed to fill a full presentation slide. Vector formats (e.g., .svg; based on mathematical equations and do not lose quality when magnified) are preferable to raster formats (e.g., .jpg; based on pixels and lose quality when magnified).

Panels Panels can consolidate related findings and help navigate figure limits. For example, a single figure could comprise four figures across panels A–D. However, only combine figures that depict a single conceptual message (e.g., related subgroup analyses).

Tables

Tables often display structured data such as study population characteristics or statistical model outputs. Below are considerations for designing effective tables:

Cell spacing Match column widths to their content. Avoid wide empty columns or cramped text that unnecessarily span multiple lines. In portrait orientation, optimal column spacing should minimize the table length.

Descriptor column Standardize typeface, size, style, and capitalization. Left alignment is typically aesthetic. Fonts should be legible without magnification. Indent subcategories under broader descriptors. Specify summary measures (e.g., No [%], median [IQR], mean [SD]). If summary measures vary throughout rows, specify them next to each descriptor.

Data column Standardize typeface, size, and style. Center alignment is typically aesthetic. Present numbers using consistent decimal places. If journals do not offer guidance, follow discipline-specific norms (e.g., one decimal place is typically sufficient for health services research).

Hypothesis tests Most baseline tables do not concern hypothesis testing. When hypothesis testing is involved, the exact P-value should be recorded (e.g., $P = 0.024$, not $P < 0.05$). If journals do not offer guidance, a common practice is to report two decimal places for $P \geq 0.01$, three decimal places for $0.001 \leq P < 0.01$, and $P < 0.001$ for smaller values.

Below is a hypothetical example of a suboptimal table, followed by opportunities for improvement and a revised table.

Suboptimal Table Example (Table 9.1)

Table 9.1 Demographic characteristics

	OP group	NOP group	*P* value
Female	32%	22%	0.04
Male	68%	78%	0.04
Age	*32 (30–36)*	*46 (40–49)*	<0.05
Race			<0.05
American Indian or Alaska Native	13%	11%	
Asian	15%	12%	
Black or African American	12%	15%	
Native Hawaiian or Other Pacific Islander	18%	28%	
White	42%	34%	
Alcohol use	3%	2%	0.06
HLOS	*5 (7–9)*	*3 (2–4)*	<0.05
Aspirin use	12	6	0.56
ICU admission	3	1.2	<0.05
Mortality	0.49	0.12	<0.05

Opportunities for Improvement

Vague title the table is not standalone.

Unclear acronyms (OP, NOP, HLOS, ICU) Acronyms, even if described in the main text, should be described in table footnotes. Nonessential, nonuniversal acronyms should be avoided.

Duplicative content In this table, presenting the proportion of females and males is duplicative.

Illogical data presentation Baseline descriptors (e.g., alcohol use, aspirin use) and outcomes (HLOS, ICU admission) are mixed.

Unspecified summary measures and data Some summary measures (e.g., age, HLOS, ICU admission) are not specified. The exact counts should be presented in addition to percentages.

Non-intentional spacing The spacing of columns does not appear intentional.

Inconsistent decimal places Data are presented using inconsistent decimal places.

Unnecessary *P*-values *P*-values are not necessary for descriptive tables. Even if they were, exact *P*-values should be described, rather than "$P < 0.05$."

Revised Table Example (Table 9.2)

Table 9.2 Characteristics of adults at a community hospital who did and did not undergo operative management for appendicitis, 2020–2022

	Operative management $N = 986$	Nonoperative management $N = 823$
Female, *No. (%)*	316 (32)	181 (22)
Age, *median (IQR)*, years	32 (30–36)	46 (40–49)
Race, *No. (%)*		
American Indian or Alaska Native	128 (13)	91 (11)
Asian	148 (15)	99 (12)
Black or African American	118 (12)	123 (15)
Native Hawaiian or other Pacific Islander	177 (18)	230 (28)
White	415 (42)	280 (34)
Alcohol use, *No. (%)*	30 (3)	16 (2)
Aspirin use, *No. (%)*	118 (12)	49 (6)
Hospital length of stay, *median (IQR)*, days	5 (7–9)	3 (2–4)
ICU admission, *No. (%)*	30 (3)	10 (1)
Inpatient mortality, *No. (%)*	5 (0.5)	1 (0.1)

Acronyms: *ICU* intensive care unit

Chapter 10
The Discussion and Conclusion: After the Story

A well-written Introduction explains *why* a study is important and its aim; a well-written Methods explains *how* the aim was investigated; and a well-written Results presents *facts* that speak for themselves. By the end of the Results, readers will already have derived their own conclusions. If your study was designed and communicated well, these should match your own. Many fear writing the *Discussion*, but the hard work is done. The Discussion simply walks readers through the final stretch toward the inevitable: your one key message.

Ibrahim and Dimick's "*Writing for Impact*" chapter outlines an intuitive formula for this stretch, on which I will build: summarize the facts, highlight how your findings fill the critical knowledge gap, present actionable next steps, and disclose and contextualize limitations.

Summarize the Facts

The Results presented a series of facts, including tables, figures, descriptive statistics, and analytic outcomes. The first paragraph of the *Discussion* should provide a birds-eye narrative of these findings centered on the study aim and hypothesis. Do not re-list the facts. Rather, consider this paragraph as the one-paragraph movie review: not a scene-by-scene recap, but the critic's main takeaways.

A practical tip is to first copy the last paragraph of your Introduction (*"We aimed to....we hypothesized that..."*). Next, add several sentences that explain how your study achieved the aim and whether your hypothesis was supported. You don't have to recount every secondary analysis. Recall the one key message of your study; what sequence of findings would lead readers to realize the same conclusion on their own? Often, general descriptions (e.g., all, most, a majority) suffice, rather than precise statistics. At the end, delete the sentences copied from the *Introduction*.

J. Choi, *The Research Publishing Playbook*,
https://doi.org/10.1007/978-3-032-28504-1_10

What remains is your first Discussion paragraph: a natural summary of your study's findings.

If a manuscript were a children's book, the Introduction ended with "a long, long, time ago." The Methods and Results completed the story. With the Discussion, you are closing the book, spending a minute to recap, and sharing the story's lessons with eager listeners.

Highlight How Your Findings Fill a Critical Knowledge Gap

The Introduction's second paragraph defined the urgent and critical knowledge gap. The next section of your Discussion should directly answer whether and how your study filled this gap.

As with the summary paragraph, begin by copying your *Introduction* sentences that describe the knowledge gap. Use this as a visual scaffold to ensure your paragraph centers on the gap and how your study filled this gap. After deleting the copied text, what remains will be a convincing narrative that presents your study's added value to the literature.

The Introduction provided a broad overview of the knowledge gap, and this is the time to discuss the close-up details:

What did prior studies find, and why was the gap unresolved?
Did previous limitations involve the study population, study design, or analysis?

Remember to maintain a professional and measured tone when reviewing prior studies; their authors could be your reviewers. Rather than criticizing, factually discuss what was and was not explored.

After detailing the gap, walk readers through exactly how your findings filled the gap:

Did you study the question in a unique population or setting?
Did you design the study to facilitate more robust inference?
What was truly unique about your study, that it answered a question that was unknown?

Remember—readers only know what you write. What may be obvious to you should not be assumed for your readers. Spell out why your study adds value and re-iterate why the gap mattered in the first place.

Among many potential prior studies to discuss, a practical strategy is to cite the most contemporary studies published in the most widely recognized journals. Reviewers and readers are human, and the halo effect is unavoidable. A study that cites contemporary and reputable references will signal that it concerns current and important questions. Make sure to read every reference you cite, beyond the title and abstract. Every cited fact should be directly traceable in the referenced study.

Present Actionable Next Steps

Communicating your study's importance should be balanced with acknowledging that a single study rarely offers the final word. Before the Conclusion, an action plan should outline how we can deepen understanding.

For a retrospective study, avoid the generic "*prospective study is needed to verify these findings*." Researchers rarely follow up with a prospective study and not every question can be answered in prospective fashion. What can be addressed in the meantime? If your study was designed to be hypothesis-generating, detail how the follow-up study should be designed and to what end—why is more study needed? Rather than suggesting more study for the sake of more study, a thoughtful agenda should be outlined. If your study has immediate implications for understanding, practice, or policy, these should be discussed.

Align the strength of your recommendations with the strength of your evidence. Overstatements undermine credibility. On the other hand, failure to provide actionable next steps undermines impact.

Limitations: Disclose and Contextualize

The limitations paragraph is one of the most important components in the manuscript. Reviewers will use this to gauge whether investigators designed a study thoughtfully, employed rigorous analyses, and drew logical conclusions based on objective assessment of findings. Most limitations are methodological. A strong paragraph must disclose all limitations and contextualize how they were mitigated or why claims remain valid.

A useful framework is a 2 × 2 grid of predictability (whether a limitation could have been foreseen) and addressability (whether a limitation could be mitigated with reasonable resources; Fig. 10.1).

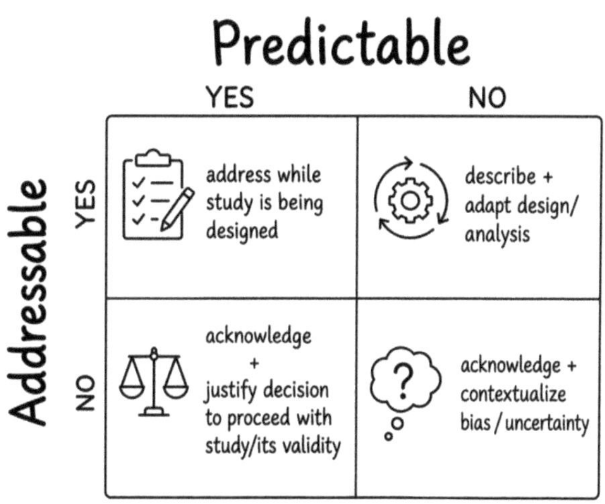

Fig. 10.1 A framework to classify and pre-emptively address study limitations

Predictable and addressable limitations should not appear because they should have been addressed before the study began. Involving an expert methodologist early reduces the risk of a reviewer pointing out an obvious oversight. If you notice this limitation, address it before submission. For example, rather than stating that the study's validity under an alternative model assumption is unclear, conduct the sensitivity analysis.

Predictable and unaddressable limitations often stem from structural constraints of data, study design, or available resources. For example, all databases have inherent limitations; many questions must be explored retrospectively before warranting prospective, experimental study; a research group may lack resources to employ the most advanced tools. Acknowledge these limitations and their potential impact on findings directly, and ensure your tone, conclusions, and target journals reflect these limitations. Beyond acknowledgement, justify the decision to proceed with the study (e.g. *"although the database has *** gaps, it remains most appropriate resource to answer this question for *** reasons*").

Unpredictable and addressable limitations include external disruptions that investigators could not have foreseen but could reasonably adapt to. For example, a hospital's lab assay platform or relevant policies may change mid-study, and a site in a multicenter study may drop out. Describe such disruptions and how a study design or analysis was adapted to preserve validity. Sudden disruptions sometimes can reframe studies as natural experiments, creating opportunities for instrumental variable analysis.

Unpredictable and unaddressable limitations are events investigators could not have foreseen or reasonably corrected. For example, a pandemic may halt enrollment for long periods. These simply need to be acknowledged. If possible, explain the suspected direction of bias or degree of uncertainty. Even if uncorrectable, transparent contextualization shows thoughtful scholarship.

Pitfalls

One principle can guard against most pitfalls in the Discussion: stay humble and stick to logic and common sense. Reviewers and readers have no personal investment in your study. They will evaluate facts and whether your interpretations align with the evidence. It is natural to believe strongly in the importance of one's study, overstate its significance, or be attached to the original hypothesis, but these subconscious biases can sway the narrative away from what the data support. Stay humble—acknowledge that most studies are incremental. Stay impartial— interpret findings through the lens of logic and common sense.

The Conclusion

With the Discussion complete, the Conclusion distills everything into one final message. This is the last chance to deliver your one takeaway. Four sentences can structure a memorable ending:

First, summarize the findings; one concise sentence.
Second, state the implications; this is your takeaway.
Third, show humility; highlight a limitation or safeguard against overly optimistic interpretations.
Last, end with a call to action.

A disciplined Conclusion should leave readers with a takeaway that feels both justified and inevitable.

Part III
After the Writing

Chapter 11
Reviewing Your Manuscript: Be Your Toughest Critic

Congratulations—your draft is complete! Now, set it aside for at least 1 week before starting revisions. Do not immediately review your draft. Do not think about your study. Effective revision requires impartiality. Time away is mandatory to separate emotionally and intellectually from the study you devoted months or years, crafting. Errors that were blurred from subconsciously skipping familiar writing will be more apparent after a week-long break. If you are writing toward a submission deadline, set your internal deadline at least 2 weeks before the actual deadline.

This chapter outlines strategies for reviewing as the first author, then additional guidance for reviewing as a principal investigator and a coauthor.

Reviewing as the First Author

Do not circulate writing you are not proud of. Your team entrusted you to take this study to the finish line, and the writing is your key responsibility. Even if a team allocates writing among coauthors, ultimately, it is the first author's responsibility to piece the sections together, revise, and circulate a polished draft for review.

Obvious spelling and grammatical errors, poorly formatted tables, and sloppy writing hurt your reputation as a researcher among your peers and mentors. Guard the manuscript from leaving your inbox until every word and inch has been reviewed. Consider the following three-pass strategy to ensure every circulated draft is polished.

1. The "content" pass: understand the big picture.

After a week-long break, the manuscript should feel unfamiliar enough for a fresh read. On your first pass, read the manuscript from the perspective of a *topic-naive reader* from the beginning to the end. Focus on major issues using the following checklist (Table 11.1); don't linger on every spelling error.

J. Choi, *The Research Publishing Playbook*,
https://doi.org/10.1007/978-3-032-28504-1_11

Table 11.1 A checklist to identify major errors during first-pass manuscript review

Does the introduction present a clear knowledge gap and study aim?
Are the methods easy to understand and logically presented?
Were all analyses essential for the study aim conducted?
Are results presented in the same order as the methods?
Are results factual, without editorializing?
Are figures and tables of presentable quality, essential, and standalone?
Are interpretations proportional to the data, without overstatement?
Is the knowledge gap, and how findings filled this gap, clear?
Is a logical action plan or implication outlined?
Are all limitations acknowledged and thoughtfully discussed?
Is the key takeaway unmistakable?

Revise the manuscript until every item on this checklist can be answered with an unequivocal *Yes*. By the end of this pass, the manuscript should contain all components necessary for a polished draft.

2. The "style" pass: read every word out loud.

For the second pass, read every word out loud. We have a tendency to skip words and sentences when "visually reading" the manuscript out of familiarity. Reading aloud simulates what reviewers or readers will be "hearing" when they read your manuscript for the first time.

Listen from the perspective of your grade-school English teacher. This is the pass that ensures concise, clear communication. Any sentence that sounds awkward should be rewritten. Any sentence that forces a breath or loses its logical thread is too long and should be split. At each level, interrogate necessity:

Sentence: is every word essential?
Paragraph: is every sentence essential?
Section: is every paragraph essential?

Eliminate any filler words and redundant ideas. Use the active voice and punctuation strategically (colons, semicolons, em dashes) to tighten prose. When possible, use the Supplement to keep Methods or Results in the main text more concise.

By the end of this pass, every word should have a purpose and the manuscript should flow clearly. Most first drafts can be reduced by roughly one-third at this stage.

3. The "ruthless" pass: critique with all your might.

For your third pass, become a ruthless critic. Challenge every logic, scan every inch of figures, and hunt for every possible error. Imagine that you will be rewarded for every error you find. Read every word in the manuscript again from the title onward, using this checklist (Table 11.2).

After addressing every identifiable error, take at least 1 day off, then re-read the manuscript as a ruthless reviewer. Repeat until no errors are detected.

At this point, the draft is ready for circulation to the principal investigator, then the coauthors. Many principal investigators will request to review before the draft is circulated to the full team.

Table 11.2 A detailed checklist to identify errors during final-pass manuscript review

Is the title or abstract misleading or overstated?
Does the title employ strategic keywords?
Does every sentence flow without logic gaps?
Is the presented knowledge gap genuine or a product of incomplete literature review?
Is the study aim really meaningful?
Did any methods employ common pitfalls?
Does an expert methodologist agree there are no errors?
Do all reported results correspond to analyses planned in the Methods?
Are all fonts, spacings, and graphical elements in figures/tables readable and intentional?
Do all numbers in tables and figures add up correctly where relevant?
Are all claims supported by presented findings, given the limitations?
Are there any limitations that were not disclosed?
Is every limitation contextualized logically?
Is every referenced fact directly traceable to the cited source?
Does the manuscript fully adhere to the journal formatting guideline?

Reviewing as the Principal Investigator

Ideally, your first author (who has read this book) sends a polished draft that requires little revision. In reality, every principal investigator has stylistic preferences and knows discipline-specific expectations that may not appear in general writing advice. Each revision round between the first author and principal investigator delays progress, because at least one party will have competing commitments that bar immediate response. The goal should be to pre-emptively minimize the number of revision iterations.

Set clear expectations with your first author about when you want to see drafts. Experienced first authors may be ready to send only the polished version. Others may benefit from earlier feedback after completing individual sections. Whatever your preference, share examples of what you consider high-quality writing (e.g., specific articles, journals) to set explicit standards. Early expectation-setting can obviate many revision rounds.

If you find yourself red-lining most of a draft, stop. Do not rewrite the entire manuscript. Allow your mentee the opportunity to learn and revise independently. Moreover, rewriting a full manuscript is often a suboptimal use of your time. A more efficient approach is a brief live-edit session, where you demonstrate common errors, specify sections that need major revision, and clarify expectations. Live-edit a portion of the manuscript and ask your trainee to adapt for the remainder of the manuscript. Fifteen to thirty minutes of live editing can often replace hours of asynchronous revisions. If this book has been useful, share it with your trainees and ask them to follow the guidance.

Once you are satisfied with the draft, circulate it to coauthors with a firm deadline. Coauthors should provide suggestions within that window or be assumed to have none. While waiting for every individual schedule may feel courteous, engaged coauthors should not be surprised by the submission schedule. In most cases, a 1-week window is sufficient.

Reviewing as a Coauthor

Be a responsible colleague and provide feedback. Your name will be tied to the published work permanently, so ensure you agree with all content. Respect the principal investigator's role; line-level edits are usually unnecessary, and your stylistic preferences should not dominate. Focus your comments on substantive issues. If you truly do not see a need for revision, affirm this explicitly rather than remaining silent.

Chapter 12
The Cover Letter to Survive the Editor's Desk

There is only one chance to make a first impression. When a manuscript is submitted, the editor will typically review the cover letter and abstract—and perhaps, select sections of the manuscript—before deciding whether to desk reject or send the manuscript out for peer review. To survive the editor's desk, the cover letter must convince the editor of two things:

The study will interest the journal's audience.
The study meets the journal's standards for quality.

Editors will typically review submissions in batches and often, during brief windows between obligations. Your cover letter must be strategically designed to achieve these two goals quickly. Like every other part of a manuscript, a refined template should be used for every cover letter.

Header

The header is an opportunity to signal your brand. If you are part of an established group that regularly publishes in the journal or a well-recognized department in the domain, display the logo prominently. This instantly cues familiarity and credibility.

Introduction

Address the letter to the editor-in-chief or simply to "editors". You often cannot predict which editor will triage your submission, and none will take offense at a general greeting. If resubmitting to a different journal, do remember to make appropriate edits to your cover letter.

J. Choi, *The Research Publishing Playbook*,
https://doi.org/10.1007/978-3-032-28504-1_12

A well-designed study title is itself an opportunity to broadcast the study's interest to the journal audience. Place the study title immediately after the greeting, in bold font:

Dear Dr. *editor-in-chief's last name* or Dear Editors,

Re: [STUDY TITLE]

Body

Open with a direct statement:

We wish to submit the manuscript as an [article type]

This classifies expectations immediately. This is especially important for non-original investigations (e.g., editorial, short letter, review article), as editors will be primed to have specific expectations when reviewing the cover letter or abstract. For example, a review article typically attracts many citations, and the editor will subconsciously look for cues that your topic would interest the audience and drive readership.

Next, **establish the importance of the topic and the knowledge gap.** In a few sentences, demonstrate why the topic matters to the journal's audience and highlight the critical and urgent knowledge gap. The editor must believe that:

the topic is timely and important;
the gap is real;
and a well-executed study addressing the gap would be meaningful and attract broad readership.

Afterwards, **summarize how the study filled the knowledge gap, emphasize rigor, and implications of findings**. Avoid excessive numerical detail (e.g., confidence intervals). Use keywords that emphasize the study's methodologic rigor. Show the editor why the findings matter and articulate how the findings advance the field.

Closing

After priming the editors, end with a deliberate statement:

We believe this study will be well-read by your readership including ***, and will make important contributions for ***.

Thank the editor for their time.

The signature is your last opportunity to signal expertise. List key authors whose reputation will strengthen the submission, and their titles. This typically includes the principal investigator and select co-authors.

OLIVE OIL health consortium

Dear Editors,

Re: A Randomized Controlled Trial Evaluating the Efficacy of Olive Oil for Mitigating Symptoms of the Common Cold

We wish to submit this manuscript as an *Original Article.*

The common cold remains one of the most frequent causes of outpatient visits worldwide, yet evidence-based options for symptomatic relief remain limited. Although a wide range of home remedies are commonly used, existing evidence supporting these interventions is largely anecdotal or observational, with few adequately powered randomized trials evaluating patient-centered outcomes. As a result, clinicians and patients lack reliable data to guide self-directed, low-cost symptom management.

We conducted a **multicenter, double-blind randomized controlled trial** enrolling 1,204 adults with new-onset upper respiratory symptoms. Participants were assigned to daily supplementation with extra-virgin olive oil or placebo for five days. Compared with placebo, the olive-oil group experienced a **32% reduction in symptom-severity**, a **shorter median illness duration**, and **fewer subsequent clinical encounters for symptom progression**. Adherence exceeded 90%, and findings were consistent across prespecified subgroups and sensitivity analyses.

To our knowledge, this study provides the first adequately powered experimental evidence evaluating a widely accessible dietary intervention for common-cold symptom mitigation. Given the substantial global burden of the common cold and practicality of this intervention, we believe these results will be of broad interest to the *World Journal of Primary Care's* readership, including primary care physicians, implementation researchers, and the lay public.

Thank you in advance for your time and consideration.

Sincerely,

Alexandra Johnson, MD, MPH
Principal Investigator
Chair of Olive Oil Health Consortium

Daniel Lee, PhD
Associate Professor of Biostatistics

Jane Raman, MD
Professor of Otolaryngology
Vice Chair of Research, Department of Otolaryngology

Fig. 12.1 Example of an effective cover letter

Every word in the cover letter, including the signature line, should be deliberate. Use the fewest possible words. Including institutional logos and signatures, the letter should not exceed one page. Figure 12.1 presents an example of an effective cover letter.

A successful cover letter should leave the editor feeling eager to read the abstract, convinced that the study addresses an important problem that will interest the journal's audience and exceeds the journal's quality standards. A cover letter is much more than a formality; it is a strategic tool for clearing the first gate toward publication.

Chapter 13
Responding to Reviewers, Including Reviewer #2

Receiving a request for revision means your manuscript has cleared a major milestone: the editor has decided the study is potentially publishable and worth additional consideration. Cognitively, it is important to recognize the reality that most revision decisions —especially major revisions—are closer to "rejection" than "acceptance." In many cases, rescuing the manuscript requires considerable effort. Recall that in the journey of a research study from its conception to publication, the submission is approximately the halfway point. Whether the second half of this journey is considerably shorter or longer will depend on reviewers' comments and how you craft your responses.

How Editors Interpret Reviewer Recommendations

After manuscripts pass the editor's desk, most journals seek at least two independent reviewers' input before editors make the next decision. The Table 13.1 summarizes typical editorial tendencies based on the permutation of these reviewers' recommendations.

Many manuscripts returned for revisions will fall into the bolded scenarios, where at least one reviewer recommended a major revision. Even when a revision opportunity is offered, the ultimate decision will likely be a rejection unless reviewer concerns are convincingly addressed. When given a revision opportunity, your task is to eliminate any reason for the editor or reviewers to ultimately reject the manuscript.

J. Choi, *The Research Publishing Playbook*,
https://doi.org/10.1007/978-3-032-28504-1_13

Table 13.1 Typical editorial tendencies based on reviewer recommendations

Typical outcome	Reviewer #1	Reviewer #2
Accept	Accept	Accept
Accept with minor revision	Accept	Minor revision
Accept with minor revision	Minor revision	Minor revision
Revision > reject	**Major revision**	**Minor revision**
Reject ~ revision	**Major revision**	**Major revision**
Reject >> revision	**Major revision**	**Reject**
Reject	Reject	Reject

Read the Room

Before drafting any response, the first task is to read between the lines and grasp each reviewer's *general stance* and *primary concerns*.

General stances include supportive, unimpressed, skeptical, and highly critical. Characterizing the general stance can guide an overall strategy for the response:

Supportive: avoid introducing new concerns. Respond succinctly and directly. Make only the requested changes.

Unimpressed: better communicate why the study matters. Clarify the knowledge gap and reframe why the question was worth answering. Explicitly state the study's contribution.

Skeptical: demonstrate methodologic and analytic rigor. Respond with structured, evidence-based explanations, clarifying design choices and assumptions.

Highly critical: respond using measured, professional language. Address valid concerns and, when needed, direct responses toward editorial judgment rather than reviewer appeasement.

Primary concerns typically fall into two buckets: methodological (e.g., inadequate sample size, suboptimal data set, or statistical model) and writing (e.g., overstatements, style). Write down the *one* concern per reviewer that precluded them from recommending an acceptance. Write down any common concerns among reviewers. Getting a general "read of the room" is the first step to strategize your response. Remember, the goal of your response to reviewers is to address every concern and eliminate any reason to reject your manuscript.

Adopt an Appreciative Attitude

Few authors would describe reading reviewer comments as a *pleasant* experience. However, perceiving these comments as "obstacles" to manuscript acceptance is counterproductive. Reviewers volunteer their time. They read manuscripts during their work breaks, weekends, or evenings, and share feedback that more often than not improves the science or its communication. Whenever possible, appreciate their time and the opportunity to craft a stronger manuscript (i.e., start each response with, "*we thank the reviewer,*" "*we appreciate the opportunity*", etc.).

Authors often view responses to reviewer comments as binary; either adopting or rejecting the suggestion. Rejecting too many suggestions, even of minor points, invites the risk of an ultimate rejection. The default response should be to adopt the reviewer's suggestion unless doing so would compromise the study's aim or scientific integrity.

Even if a suggestion must be declined, the tone of your response is as important as the substance. Do not confront or imply that the reviewer is wrong. Rather, seek every opportunity to clarify communication. Whenever there is an opportunity to revise the manuscript—even if to clarify your rationale—make the revision, rather than simply rejecting a suggestion outright. The effort to strengthen your manuscript signals goodwill and will make reviewers more receptive to your reasoning.

Approach each reviewer as a close colleague intent on strengthening your manuscript, rather than an anonymous hurdle to overcome. This mindset will make a noticeable difference in the tone of your response and could meaningfully influence the reviewer's final recommendation.

Format to Maximize Clarity

Format the response document to maximize clarity. Separate each reviewer with page breaks. Copy each reviewer's comments and break them down to individual points to address. Respond beneath each point with (1) an acknowledgement of the concern and your corrected action and (2) revised text. Avoid burying reviewers in dense paragraphs. Use standardized typography: **bold font for your response**, *italics for revised text with color/~~strikethroughs~~*.

Some reviewers start with a general review of the manuscript; these summaries do not warrant a response. If conceptually similar comments are made by the same reviewer, these may be combined into one point to answer. Consider the following comment from a reviewer:

Example Reviewer Comment

Reviewer #1 *"The authors conducted a single institution observational study evaluating the impact of *** on ***. The study population included ****. The statistical analysis comprised ***. Overall, the authors found ***. Based on these results, they conclude ***. I commend the authors for ***. *** was a great choice.*

*I have several concerns. The authors chose to exclude ***. However, this introduces the potential for ***. They defined the primary outcome using ***. Did they* *consider ***? They discuss *** but we can see the results actually show ***. They mention this limitation, but as mentioned above, excluding *** is a critical mistake."*

The first paragraph does not warrant a response. The other concerns warrant point-by-point response using standardized typography:

Example Response to Reviewer

Reviewer 1.

1. The authors chose to exclude ***. However, this introduces the potential for ***...They mention this limitation, but as mentioned above, excluding *** is a critical mistake."

   We appreciate the reviewer's point. [elaborate on response] The revised section is below:

   ****revised text in italics. **Red font to indicate new text,** ~~strikethrough~~ to indicate deleted text****
2. They defined the primary outcome using ***. Did they consider ***?

   We thank the reviewer for this insightful remark. [elaborate on response] The revised section is below:

   ****revised text in italics. **Red font to indicate new text,** ~~strikethrough~~ to indicate deleted text****
3. They discuss *** but we can see the results actually show ***.

   We agree that *. [elaborate on response]. We revised the section as *****:

   ****revised text in italics. **Red font to indicate new text,** ~~strikethrough~~ to indicate deleted text****

The 2 × 2 Framework to Respond to Reviewers

Viewing reviewer comments through a 2 × 2 framework of simplicity and reasonability helps guide the most appropriate and strategically effective response.

Simple comments demand little time or resources. These include formatting requests, minor edits to tables and figures, and straightforward analyses using data available to the group. **Challenging comments** demand considerable time or resources, such as acquiring new data or conducting complex analyses beyond the capability of the research team.

Reasonable comments are those that authors perceive would meaningfully improve the manuscript's clarity or methodologic rigor. These include points such as highlighting a methodologic weakness that undermines stated conclusions, or requesting an expanded discussion to explain why results diverge from prior literature. **Unreasonable comments** are those perceived to be unhelpful, such as unconstructive comments (e.g., "*this is just bad research*"), requests that drastically

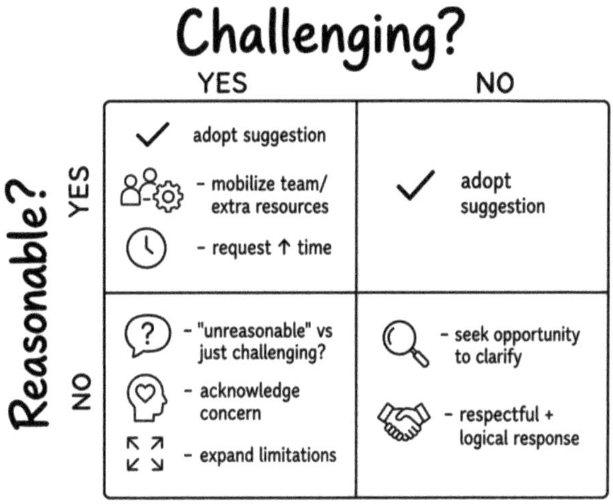

Fig. 13.1 Framework to respond to reviewer comments. Strategic responses must consider the degree of challenge required to adopt and the perceived reasonability of each suggestion

change the study direction, or factually incorrect assertions (e.g., suggestions to use statistically inappropriate methods).

The following are suggestions regarding how to respond to each comment phenotype (Fig. 13.1):

Simple and reasonable Adopt the suggestion promptly. Implement the change and thank the reviewer for the helpful recommendation.

Challenging and reasonable Adopt the suggestion. Mobilize the team or additional collaborators to respond promptly, or request additional time from the managing editor if needed to craft a thoughtful revision. Many journals provide deadlines for revisions, but these are often flexible. Do return the revision as soon as possible; reviewers will appreciate prompt turnaround while the manuscript is still fresh in their minds.

Simple and unreasonable Respond with respect and logic. Many of these comments stem from misinterpretations, which, in turn, reflect opportunities to improve communication. For example, if the reviewer misinterpreted findings, revise the corresponding section for clarity and thank the reviewer for highlighting the ambiguity.

If the comment requests simple but methodologically inappropriate changes, recognize that your goal is not to correct the reviewer (e.g., "the reviewer's suggestion is incorrect because…"). No one enjoys being corrected. Instead, recognize the opportunity to clarify your rationale. With expert guidance, explain, using supporting evidence (e.g., methodologic textbook chapter), why your approach is most appropriate and the suggested alternative may be suboptimal for the study aim. Revise your manuscript to make this rationale explicit, and thank the reviewer for the opportunity to better explain your rationale.

If a comment is unconstructive (e.g., requesting citation of low-quality studies), the editor will likely recognize this as well. Respond respectfully, but do consider whether the request is a "battle worth fighting." If adopting the suggestion does not compromise the study's scientific integrity or aim, it may be reasonable to implement it to preserve goodwill and avoid unnecessary friction.

Challenging and unreasonable First, separate "challenging" from "unreasonable." Some comments feel unreasonable simply because they require substantial effort, such as complex analyses beyond your team's expertise. These requests may still be reasonable if they meaningfully strengthen the manuscript or are necessary to meet the journal's standards. Your task would be to weigh the investment needed to address this comment against the risk of rejection and having to restart the submission process with another journal. Many times, the finite investment to address the comment is better than the unpredictable alternative.

If a comment seems truly unreasonable (e.g., request for additional patient recruitment that would take years), these concerns often reflect deeper concerns: (1) the reviewer does not see a meaningful knowledge gap the study fills, or (2) perceives a major study design limitation that was not adequately discussed. Address both concerns. Improve communicating the knowledge gap, clarify your study aim, and explain how your study design and findings addressed the gap despite its limitations. Expand the *Limitations* to acknowledge the reviewer's concern and articulate why your findings still meaningfully contribute to the literature. In your response, acknowledge the reviewer's underlying concern and revise the manuscript wherever possible to improve clarity. A respectful, well-reasoned response, paired with manuscript revisions that acknowledge the reviewer's concern, maximizes the chance of a favorable recommendation even when the specific request is not fulfilled.

Turnaround Time

Return the revision as soon as possible. Fast turnarounds offer several advantages:

1. Reviewers still remember the manuscript and their specific concerns, reducing the likelihood of identifying new concerns.
2. It signals professionalism and respect for the reviewer's time.
3. It shortens the overall time to acceptance.

Delays often force reviewers to reread the entire manuscript, increasing their workload and scrutiny. The principal investigator should set clear expectations with the team in advance, especially the first author, regarding the importance of responding promptly and the possibility of substantial revision demands. Many journals publish typical turnaround times; these should be considered when planning the team's bandwidth for revisions.

Responding to reviewers is much more than a technical exercise. It is a strategic negotiation that should be shaped by a respectful tone, clear communication, and the effort to strengthen your manuscript. Beyond factual right versus wrong, many decisions hinge on reviewers' perception of authors' effort, professionalism and responsiveness. Craft responses that give reviewers every reason to say "accept."

Afterword

Refining productive habits, building effective teams, identifying meaningful questions, conducting rigorous research, and communicating findings convincingly—the *process* of taking a research idea to peer-reviewed publication—is a distinct skill set that requires deliberate practice. Too often, these skills are acquired gradually through serendipitous mentorship or prematurely abandoned when early obstacles lead us to conclude that we were simply not "cut out for research."

I believe that anyone committed to asking important questions and willing to do the work can learn how to be an effective researcher. This book was written to accelerate the process of taking a research study from conception to the finish line so that less time is spent navigating avoidable obstacles and more time is devoted to mentoring others and thoughtfully designing and investigating studies that matter.

I continue to learn from my mentors and mentees every day. To all my mentors and mentees, past, present, and future—thank you for shaping the lessons within *The Research Publishing Playbook.*

J. Choi, *The Research Publishing Playbook*,
https://doi.org/10.1007/978-3-032-28504-1

MIX
Papier aus verantwortungsvollen Quellen
Paper from responsible sources
FSC® C105338

If you have any concerns about our products,
you can contact us on
ProductSafety@springernature.com

In case Publisher is established outside the EU,
the EU authorized representative is:
Springer Nature Customer Service Center GmbH
Europaplatz 3, 69115 Heidelberg, Germany

Printed by Libri Plureos GmbH
in Hamburg, Germany